American Medical Association
Physicians dedicated to the health of America

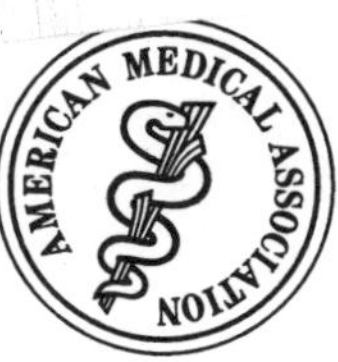

Integration Strategies for the Medical Practice

*The Physician's Handbook
to Integration Alternatives*

Editor: .... Kay Stanley
Project Assistant: .... Bonnie Cole
Author: .... Anne M. Renz
Art Director: .... Jeff Weir

Published by:

*Coker Publishing, LLC —
3150 Holcomb Bridge Road, Suite 200
Norcross, Georgia 30071
(770) 242-0118*

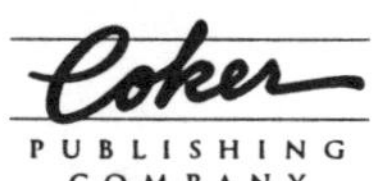

PUBLISHING
COMPANY

ISBN 0-89970-789-0

American Medical Association Preface ___________

This book and the others contained in the *PRACTICE SUCCESS!©* Series are designed to offer you concrete, practical information on topics that you may sometimes consider the least important aspect of the profession of medicine: the business of running a medical practice. And in some ways that's how it should be. The long, hard years you dedicated to medical school and residency training were meant to make you an excellent physician, not an excellent businessperson. Caring for patients is and always will be your first priority. But you cannot successfully run a medical practice without planning and without consideration of important business issues. While it takes a minimum of ten years for a person to become a physician, the day a practice opens is the day a physician becomes a small businessperson.

Your many years of superb education probably did not include much information on medical office operations, personnel management, accounting or business law. Yet these business issues are more important than ever before, because the practice of medicine in today's rapidly changing environment is far more complex than ever before. Good business management today is essential to good medical practice. The physician who ignores basic business principles in operating his or her practice may soon find that they face difficulties with suppliers, employees, the government or even their patients.

Other pressures today force physicians to search for more efficient ways of running their practices. Most physicians find demands on their time increasing tremendously. There is a daily struggle to build a practice that will earn a steady income, to schedule regular working hours, to deliver quality care to patients and to still have time for relaxation and family.

Developing an efficient practice that runs smoothly makes all of these goals attainable. The application of good business planning will enable you to spend more time on those things that are most important to you.

This book and the others in the *PRACTICE SUCCESS!©* Series are guides to medical practice management for the new physician and the established physician who wants to survey his or her practice with an eye toward improvement. These books will not provide you with solutions to every challenge that may arise in day-to-day practice. Our goal is to acquaint you with essential business principles and tools, as well as with some new approaches to managing your practice. The knowledge you acquire from this series can be supplemented by information you gather from talking with your colleagues and advisors. You will then be in a position to explore those ideas that promise to achieve the best results for your particular practice situation.

By providing the information in this book and others, the **American Medical Association (AMA)** is not endorsing any one management philosophy or method of delivering health care services. No one approach will meet the objectives of all physicians. Physicians and their staffs will have to decide for themselves what is the best way to manage their individual practices. This guide is published by the American Medical Association for educational purposes only. It is intended solely to provide general information on managed care to assist physicians in making decisions.

It is not intended to constitute legal advice and should not be relied on as a source of legal advice. If legal advice is desired or needed, a licensed attorney should be consulted. Finally, this book does not enunciate **AMA** policy. The annual *Policy Compendium* of the **AMA** sets forth our positions on such issues as contracting, policy, medical ethics, managed care and practice management.

We hope that this publication will be useful to you.

The American Medical Association

About The Coker Group

The Coker Group is a national provider of health care consultative and management services assisting physicians, hospitals, and health care systems to better position themselves to be successful in a reformed health care environment. The Coker Group offers the following services for its clients:

Programs and Services:

- Primary Care Physician Network Development

- Practice Valuations and Acquisition Negotiations

- Physician Employment and Compensation Contract Design

- The Facilitation of Group Practice Development

- Physician Practice Management Services

- Management Services Organization (MSO) Development

- Market Share Management Program

- Newly Recruited Physician Services

- Educational Programs

- Evaluation and Consultant Services

- Personnel Productivity Programs

- *PRACTICE SUCCESS!*© and *PRACTICE SUCCESS!*© Series

For more information, contact:

THE **Coker** GROUP

National Consultants to Healthcare Providers

The Coker Group / 3150 Holcomb Bridge Road / Suite 200
Norcross, Georgia 30071 / (770) 242-0118

About The Book

Integration Strategies for the Medical Practice — The Physician's Handbook to Integration Alternatives serves as a guide to navigating complex integration mechanisms and options.

Managed care organizations are experiencing significant growth as the number of enrollees in these plans climbs to more than fifty million people. Their impact on physicians practicing medicine today is unparalleled. MCO development and the general economic pressure placed on physicians have changed the way medicine is practiced. A major concern often voiced by physicians is this: "How do I position myself, as a business person within the health care industry, to ensure financial viability?"

Physicians are realizing that being a solo practitioner is extremely difficult. A myriad of new organizational models are in place all offering the potential of a secure future for the practitioner. As physicians attempt to consolidate and integrate, they are seeking the following:

- economies of scale

- access to capital

- leverage in negotiating managed care contracts

- elimination of the "headaches" of running a "business."

These changes cause physicians stress and anxiety as they look at models such as group practice(s), IPAs, MSOs, PHOs, etc., and deciding if they want to be employed, be equity partners, or look at another organizational derivative.

The information contained in *Integration Strategies for the Medical Practice* is meant to provide physicians and others with the basic tools necessary to survive and thrive in managed care markets. It combines information from a variety of sources and regions of the country. This information should serve as a supplemental guideline only and is not meant to substitute for the advice of an attorney, business or financial planner.

Integration Strategies for the Medical Practice will help the reader in the following areas:

- Discerning the changing health care environment
- Comprehending physician-hospital relationships
- Identifying physician-physician relationships
- Accepting nonproviders as physician organizers
- Providing coping tools for all physicians

Who should read this book?

This book is a direct, single-topic guide to understanding managed care for those involved in the "business side of medicine," including:

- practicing physicians
- owners of medical practices and clinics
- practice administrators and managers
- business managers of any medical business
- business administrators in health care facilities, nursing homes, or health agencies

What information can the reader find?

The reader will find practical and specific information for decision strategies for the medical practice, including:

- What is happening in other areas of the country? In what evolution stage is my practice's market?
- How do patients, members, and employer purchaser requirements fit with physician requirements?
- How do hospitals "think" and what are their strategies?
- What are the legal barriers to physician-hospital alliances? What organizational models allow their partnership?
- Who is acquiring whom and where?
- If I join a network, what do I want from it? What questions do I ask to protect my interest?
- How can physicians form successful independent networks?
- Who are the nonprovider physician organizers and what do they offer?
- What are the necessary tools to function in the integrated environment?
- What are the strengths and weakness of my practice?
- Who is a good partner for me?

How technical is the writing?

Physician Integration Strategies for the Medical Practice is written in an informal, practical style. Few terms in this book are not found regularly in a newspaper, and no discussions would appear out-of-place in a business memorandum. This publication is a nontechnical discussion about the business side of medical practice management.

Physician Integration Strategies for the Medical Practice is derived from a 500 + page medical practice management resource titled *PRACTICE SUCCESS!©* Introduced in 1993, this textbook has ongoing updates and enhancements. As publishers, we are committed to providing the most current information concerning topics of interest for the "business side of medicine." For more information on this and other resources available, contact the following:

Coker Publishing, LLC
3150 Holcomb Bridge Road
Suite 200
Norcross, GA 30071
(770) 242-0118

Managing Editor
Kay Stanley

About the Author

Anne M. Renz is Vice President, Human Resources and Administration, Professional Services Group, Allina Health System, Minneapolis, Minnesota. Ms. Renz has been active in the health care field for more than twenty years, beginning her career as a Registered Nurse. She has twice served as a hospital CEO, for ten years of her career, actively guided a hospital merger and held a variety of administrative positions in predecessor organizations to the Allina Health System. Her current role involves providing administration for the Professional Services Group of the Allina Health System which provides the linkage between physicians and the System and houses the departments of Graduate Medical Education, Continuing Medical Education, Physician Recruitment, Medical Policy, Physician Support Services, Research, Telemedicine and the Allina Medical Group. In addition, she serves as the senior human resources executive to all of Allina's 50 + clinics and its employed complement of greater than 500 providers.

A national speaker and author of several articles, and a contributor to *Managing Managed Care in the Medical Practice*, Ms. Renz also provides occasional consulting services in the areas of physician recruitment, managed care issues and multiple administrative concerns.

Overview

Integration Strategies for the Medical Practice is a response to current trends in health care. This book is written to help you, the physician, make positioning decisions for your practice. We will inform you of what is happening in many parts of the country and what doctors are doing to cope with the reality of managed care. The emerging question is: to integrate or not to integrate? If the answer is yes, by what mechanism should you choose to integrate? What options are available?

The central theme of this book is to assist physicians in exploring this ever-changing landscape and in developing strategies that will serve them now and into the future. We begin with an overview of the historical, current and future perspective on health care delivery. If we understand where we have been in the past and where we currently are, our understanding will equip us to meet the demands of the future. Changes are happening rapidly and across all geographical barriers. The database for the history is largely centered on the evolution of health care as seen through a hospital perspective. Because hospitals have been larger organizations and utilized federal funding to a greater extent, they have been tracked far longer than physician practices. As the "cottage industry" of physician practices moves into sizeable, complex business ventures, they are developing their own legacy. This legacy is now shaping the future more than ever before. Looking at the initial history is important to be able to understand the evolution of the hospital—your potential partner or competitor.

Secondly, we will look at physician–hospital relationships. Three major players comprise the managed care environment: physicians, hospitals, and payers. The sometimes awkward interplay of these institutions can create tensions. The alliances that are sprouting all involve some measure of each institution trying to control its destiny. This unit will help the physician understand hospital integration strategies, hospital to hospital alliances, and organizational models for physician and hospital partnerships.

The third unit will lead the reader through physician–physician relationships. The days when starting a practice entailed little more than "hanging out a shingle" are gone in many parts of the country. Today, having a successful medical practice is serious business and may involve developing some kind of contracting organization and integrated delivery system. This takes time, expertise and money. It also takes vision, commitment, leadership and market research.

Practicing physicians may choose to align with nonprovider organizers, such as managed care organizations or practice management companies. Whether you become an employee or act as an independent contractor, there is much to know and understand about your responsibilities in the various forms of integration.

Every physician must have an understanding of the business of practice management to survive in these turbulent times. This book will help you identify the operational strengths and weakness of your practice, and know the current worth of your practice. It will also help you select the correct partner for you and your practice.

Leaders of the health care industry forecast the virtual disappearance of independent medical practices and hospitals within the next five years. Even if the predictions are inaccurate, the conversion of medical groups and hospitals from independent to integrated status poses many questions about how to function and survive.

This book will lead you through the decision-making process of integration so you will be best prepared to meet changes wrought by the future. The good news is that physicians who carefully evaluate their strategic position often experience improved financial performance, while delivering cost-effective, high quality medical services to their patients.

Table of Contents

The Changing Health Care Environment

Introduction

We all look at the future based in part on our experiences. For example, if you were practicing medicine when driving the highways included reading the Burma Shave signs, or you remember exactly where you were when you heard John F. Kennedy had been assassinated, you probably remember medicine in a more simple time. If you have begun your career in the past ten years or so, a variety of managed care issues have been part of your entire practice experience.

While you may not have a keen interest in the history of the health care environment, a working understanding of where the industry has been will serve as good background upon which to consider integration. The history of hospitals, whether or not you decide to partner with them in any manner, will serve to illustrate the evolution of their thinking. They are a major player in most communities and must be considered a strong force in the environment.

Prior to the introduction of the Medicare and Medicaid programs of the mid-1960s, most physicians practiced in solo or small practices, and they conducted business on a one-to-one basis between the doctor and the patient. The costs of health services during the early part of this century were relatively stable, and industry growth was yet to become a major market influence.

During the 1950s, health care consumed only 4.4 percent of the Gross National Product. By 1960, the rate had moved to 5.3 percent, and by 1970, concerns were being raised as the percentage climbed to 7.3 percent. Expenditures in the Medicare and Medicaid programs were showing up on the "map" and competing heavily for a larger portion of the GNP. At the same time, general inflation was rising.

The chart on the following page demonstrates the percentage of GNP growth rates from 1929 to 1995. The estimate for the year 2005 is 17.9 percent. Though the growth is substantial, it is but one factor to measure the success or failure of the system. We often hear people talk about the dramatic rise in health care costs and find ourselves compared to other countries. What we haven't factored in (primarily because it is so difficult to measure) are the public's expectations for more available health care and the outcomes we have been able to produce.

It is believed, however, regardless of that data, the costs must be better controlled or, at a minimum, better understood so the consumer can make clear choices.

Estimates are that the public pays only four cents on the dollar out of their pockets for hospital

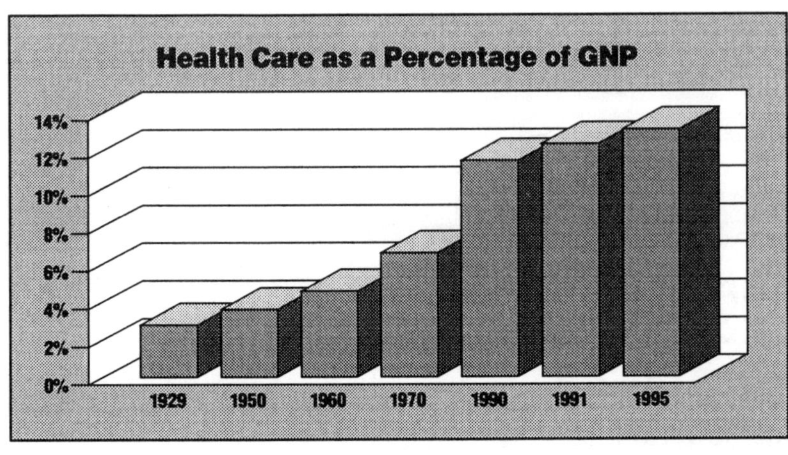

services and thirteen cents out of the dollar for physician services. The public, through its insurance vehicles, is often individually protected from feeling the economic pressures. The pressures are felt in the form of percentage of the revenues that go to pay employees' health care premiums, premium rise, taxes and the like. Studies have shown that the more people have to personally pay for their health care (i.e., actually writing a check for the services as opposed to submitting the claim to their insurance company), the more selective and prudent they become about when to seek medical care. Indeed, this is a strong argument for copayments, which are popular in the insurance industry today.

A review of major factors fueling this growth can be useful as we view our present day and attempt a reasonable forecast of the future of the health care industry.

Three major events can be held responsible for the enormous growth and the competition of health care expenditures with priorities for other goods and services within the U.S. economy.

- *Health insurance coverage became a subject of labor management negotiations.*
  Prior to the 1950s, employers did not have significant expenditures for the health care of their work force. As the demand for health insurance by the employees (and their representative unions) became a major negotiating tool, the portion of the "bottom" line employers contributed also created major influence on the profitability of many large industries. As the demand and cost of health services grew, employers began to realize even with tax advantages to the company, the expense was not sufficiently offset. Over time, we began to see the employers' coalitions that are operating in many markets today.

- *The enactment of the federally sponsored Medicare and Medicaid programs* in 1965 brought another large group into the arena. Before the introduction of these programs, 61 percent of all households paid directly for health services; business and industry paid 17 percent; and federal/state programs paid 21 percent. By 1990, we were to see that break down into approximately equal thirds. Coupled with that percentage shift, we are experiencing an aging of the population and an enormous federal deficit. The interaction of these forces has caused unprecedented pressure upon the health care system of this country.

     Chapter 1 — The Changing Health Care Environment

■ ***Technological growth*** is a major contributor to the experience and expense of those practicing and receiving services from physicians, hospitals and other providers. Before the turn of the century and the use of anesthesia, the public was more than content to live and die at home. Once surgical and antiseptic techniques began to make interventions more promising and less painful, the middle class began to seek, demand and purchase a wider variety of health care services.

Coupled with technological growth is the cost of research and development as the public began to expect/demand that science find the causes and cures for disease.

Medical Research Expenditures by Category

	1983	1993
Government	$10.778 billion	$30.828 billion
Private nonprofit agencies	456 *million*	1,248 billion
Private Industry	3.668 billion	12.254 billion

(Source: U.S. Department of Health, Education and Welfare, 1993)

The results have been astonishing reflected by improvement in perceived and real quality of life standards, numbers of procedures and cost. As an example, for those people over the age of 65, cataract surgery with lens implants, rare in 1972, was performed 3,765,000 times in 1988. Hip replacements performed a mere 25,000 times in 1972 grew to 816,000 in 1988. More than 128,500 organ transplants were performed in the eight years between 1982 and 1990.

The industry has exploded and along with it, higher demands for service and access along with less appetite for financing the costs.

Today's Environment

"The elderly shall inherit the earth," or so it seems as we begin to experience a very large group of individuals who are affluent, exert enormous political clout, consume a large quantity of government resources, are no longer in the productive work force and are continuing to experience an increase in their life expectancy. Estimates are that by 2030, persons over 65 will comprise a full 20 percent of the population.

The implications of this trend are overwhelming and will place increasing burdens on government (from which 40 percent of the elderly derive 100 percent of their income) and the health care industry. Chronic illness will consume more resources, long-term care will be a more important part of the continuum, and we will face multiple moral and ethical dilemmas as we attempt to determine the amount of resources to dedicate to a group who will have fewer years to maximize on the advantages of science and technology. We will be faced with trying to balance the demand created by sheer volume with the needs and demands of the younger, less affluent population. We are seeing increasing considerations concerning the right to die, assisted suicide and limiting care to certain age groups — difficult decisions, necessary decisions.

Nationally, we are seeing the middle class shrink, increasing numbers of women in the work force and the income distribution increasing to the top one percent of the country's population. The needs of the populations are not in keeping with their economic base. Again, health care will experience increased pressures.

The demography of the country is also experiencing an influx of immigrants, many of whom have difficulty securing work, are untrained and uneducated. Additionally, their cultures demand different medical services than those valued by the western world. Again, this increases the pressure on our system to deliver more and different services than ever before in a constrained market. Though immigrants may not have employers representing them in a block, they will require large segments of the health care dollar in the future based on sheer volume.

Through all these changes, consumers are taking a proactive role in their life and health care decisions. They are demanding partnerships in determining the type and frequency of care they receive. They are using the technology available to aid them in self-diagnosis, physician selection, payment options and the like. They have questions and demand answers.

In 1995, Allina Health System, Minneapolis, conducted an Environmental Assessment, representing a comprehensive scanning of the trends in the external environment that could have a strategic impact. Allina developed it through the assistance of a cross-company team and represented key trends in demographics and lifestyle changes, technology, industry and political/policy trends with the implications of each. A key area was to assess the requirements of the new system as expressed by patients, employers, payers and physicians. (It is noted the Minneapolis market is unique. This study should serve to demonstrate the requirements of patients, members, employer purchasing groups and physicians in a market considered mature in managed care evolution. These requirements can serve as helpful elements to consider regardless of your current market. If you are thinking about partnering with employers, health plans or systems, these drivers should be considered. As you look at your patient population, their requirements will also be of utmost importance to you in functioning in a competitive market.) The survey information follows:

Patient Requirements

- Education and communication with providers
- Respect for needs and preferences
- Provision of emotional and physical comfort
- Family involvement
- Discharge preparation
- Quality
- Access to care/availability of services
- Financing of care
- Other:
    - Recommendation from physician, nurse, family member, friend
    - Cleanliness
    - Security
    - Technology/equipment
    - Courtesy of staff
    - Responsive, reliable service

Member Requirements

- Continuity/choice of physicians*
- Access*
- Quality of care*
- Cost*
- Service/ease of use
- Coverage relative to perceived needs*
- Relevant information
- Previous level of experience with plan (satisfier, not requirement)

    Designates key requirements and expectations.

    Note: "Members" of a health plan are differentiated from "patients" in that they may or may not receive direct care and are choosing plan membership in order to accommodate their needs as patients. The difference is subtle, but one worth making.

Employer Purchaser Requirements

Health Plan

- Employee acceptance
- Continuity/choice of physicians*
- Access*
- Quality (health plan and network)
- Cost containment/managed care strategies*
- Service/ease of administration*
- Coverage
- Product design flexibility

   Designates key requirements and expectations

Implications for delivering services indicate the need for the following:

- Partnership built on shared and negotiated risk
- Single bill (integration of all care providers)
- Patient involvement/informed decision-making
- Positive experience for the patient (high level of patient satisfaction)
- Prompt return to work

   Note: Clinical quality is assumed

Physician Requirements

"Health System"

- Collaborative relationships
- Support and resources
- Patient involvement/education
- Technology/information systems
- Service quality

   Note: Not all physicians, depending upon the size and philosophy of their group and the environment in which they practice will choose to partner with a health system. For those who do, the above requirements are significant reasons why they choose to affiliate.

The delivery of services will require:

- Communication
- Collaboration

- Partnership

- Participation

Health Plans

- Increased access to capital

- Ability to further professional goals; rewards for delivery high quality care

- Control of health care delivery; autonomy

- Defend/increase patient base; increase revenue due to an increased market share

- Limited financial risk

- User-friendly systems and procedures

    Note: Just as all physicians will not choose to affiliate with a system, the level of affiliation with a health plan will vary. For those who affiliate with a health plan, the requirements above must be met to maximize the value of the affiliation.

Other parts of the country are seeing their systems being driven in new ways, as well. In Nashville, Tennessee, where Columbia/HCA has a strong presence, there is an increasing amount of collaboration between hospitals seeking to extend services outside Davidson County. The Middle Tennessee Healthcare Group, L.L.C., has been formed by Baptist Hospital, St. Thomas Hospital and Vanderbilt University Hospital. Their plans are to set up a physician network, hospitals and clinics in high growth areas, seeking relationships outside Nashville "proper" and working to build relationships with providers in these areas. Though the shadow of Columbia/HCA is a motivating force, they are also being driven by access to capital, purchasing power for supplies, securing covered lives through alliances with physicians and sharing of costs.

Houston, Texas is undergoing massive change. The system that has centered largely around the Texas Medical Center, Baylor College of Medicine and the University of Texas Medical School is now moving rapidly toward managed care. Two hospital-based networks have formed and speculation is that a third one is soon to follow. At present, only 20 percent of Houstonians belong to a gatekeeper health plan. Large numbers of physicians are practicing primary care though they are not organized in any particular fashion today. Practices are being purchased, there is a plethora of managed care plans and the mergers abound. A group of primary care physicians has formed Prime Healthcare Providers in an attempt to organize to manage risk. MetLife is in the market with more than 300,000 covered lives. The Houston Area Health Care Coalition has been formed with 56 members and a number of major employers. The market is fluid, dynamic and chaotic.

The drivers of these various markets may not be as clearly defined as they are in more mature areas like Minneapolis/St. Paul. The ones identified in the Allina study are always present— their degree of importance and the presence of many other drivers often define the difference between markets that are evolving at variable rates.

Our world and our work must change to satisfy a variety of requirements that our industry did not anticipate even two decades ago. As care givers, physicians can meet the challenges brought on by change through their individual and collaborative efforts. The new challenges cannot be addressed by repackaging the old answers. The entire industry will be called upon to manage change and the necessary transitions for change.

We will begin to explore some options available.

CHAPTER 2

Physician–Hospital Relationships

Hospital Integration Strategies

This section will explore the position of hospitals in the overall integration efforts. Though physicians will not necessarily choose to partner with hospitals, for those that do, as well as for those in leadership positions in hospitals and health systems, it is important to know the roles they are currently playing. For those choosing not to partner, a review of the strengths hospitals have and the barriers they face can be useful in the overall deliberations of whether or not to integrate with this element of the health care system. The "business" is being segmented. What is done in the hospital setting and what is done in physician offices are often areas of strong competition.

"I am called eccentric for saying in public that hospitals, if they wish to be sure of improvement:

- *Must find out what their results are*

- *Must analyze their results to find their strong and weak points*

- *Must compare their results with those of other hospitals*

- *Must care for what cases they can care for well, and avoid attempting to care for cases which they are not qualified to care for well*

- *Must welcome publicity not only for their successes, but for their errors, so that the public may give them their help when it is needed*

- *Must promote members of the medical staff on the basis which gives due consideration to what they can and do accomplish for their patients.*

Such opinions will not be eccentric a few years hence."

— E. A. Codman, M.D.
A Study in Hospital Efficiency, 1916.

To determine the most efficient way to meet the demands of the new market, hospital executives must understand their market, and the strengths, weaknesses, opportunities, threats to/of their organizations. They must be clear about the business in which they are engaged.

Traditionally, hospitals have measured the number of beds, inpatient days, average length of stays, hours per patient day and the like to gauge their progress toward profitable net revenues. They have been in the job of filling their beds, maximizing their revenue and providing a variety of inpatient and outpatient services. They have primarily defined their business based upon what they owned in visible assets—bricks and mortar, the new ER, the ambulatory surgery center, etc. With today's environment of declining reimbursement, the move away from illness and toward wellness has placed hospitals in a crisis concerning their missions, the traditional ways of doing business and their strategies for success. Organizations thrived on an old model; they continue to have reputation, identity, pride and expenses associated with those models.

Hospitals today are attempting to form partnerships or, at a minimum, loosely structured alliances with several organizations and/or services. They are emphasizing the elements of the marketplace that will meet the demands of patients and payers, i.e., preventive services and primary care.

In the past, hospital systems were built on a model of illness, specialty services, "more is better," filling beds, building new buildings, and adding technology to compete with other hospitals. This happened even if the market did not need services such as two or three CT scans in one city, more than one cancer treatment center, etc. The name of the game was to compete with the other hospitals in the market. The market was saturated in most major cities and services were duplicated at an alarming rate. In the process, these organizations incurred significant debt and added staff to support the plethora of services that were growing at an exponential rate. Hospitals have had much experience at "gearing up" and limited experience/success at "gearing down." As large, bureaucratic organizations, they have not been able to "turn on a dime," and being "nimble" was out of the question.

Hospitals outside metropolitan areas followed suit, although to a lesser degree, trying to maintain their economic strength and protect the economic base of their communities. Often, they are the largest employers (generally except governmental or school systems) in their area; they are key to the economic stability of the community.

Now, the markets (i.e., the payers) are demanding models of wellness, concerning themselves with the health of populations (not individuals), clamoring for primary care services, reducing reimbursement and spurning the "more is better" theory. Hospitals must struggle to survive from the strategies that strengthened their positions less than a decade ago.

"Partnerships will be made between groups not previously imaginable as partners. Between alternative therapies and more traditional health care. Between health care providers, insurers and communities. We'll enlarge our definition of what we're responsible for and to whom we're accountable.... Everyone's definition of results will change, moving from counting the number of beds that are filled to also counting the number of people we've kept too healthy to need one."

> — *Gordon Sprenger*
> *President, American Hospital Association*
> *Executive Officer, Allina Health System*

The American Hospital Association surveyed 6,000 hospitals and health care organizations to look at the collaborative efforts taking place in the marketplace. The 1994-1995 edition of AHA Hospital Statistics reports on 1993 data. Following is what they found:

- In keeping with the demands of the market, organizations are attempting to embrace the concepts of preventive medicine and rely more heavily on primary care networks.

- 83 percent of all hospitals provide health promotion programs.

- 60 percent of community hospitals are working with social services, public agencies or community representatives to assess the health needs of the community.

- Hospitals are increasingly providing home health care and long term care in their cadre of services.

- In the last decade, hospital inpatient days have declined 21 percent, outpatient visits have risen by 74.7 percent, and 55.4 percent of all surgeries at community hospitals were performed without overnight stays, a 21 percent increase.

- The total number of U.S. hospitals has been declining since 1977. Thirty-four community hospitals closed and 18 merged in 1993.

The chart that follows is a good indicator of some strategies hospitals are using to strengthen their positions and further their integration efforts.

Services	Owned or provided by hospital or subsidiary	Provided by hospital's system	Provided through joint ventures or similar arrangement	Provided through formal contractual or other arrangements
General acute	85.7%	5.0%	0.5%	2.2%
Intensive care	75.5%	5.1%	0.8%	5.4%
Ambulatory care	78.5%	5.1%	0.8%	5.4%
Ambulatory surgery	80.1%	5.4%	1.5%	2.7%
Emergency services	82.1%	5.1%	0.8%	6.1%
Diagnostic testing	82.2%	6.2%	3.5%	12.1%
Nursing facility	35.8%	8.0%	0.9%	12.5%
Rehab	52.0%	6.6%	1.5%	15.9%
Psychiatric	33.3%	6.9%	1.2%	20.3%
Home health	39.8%	8.8%	3.7%	23.4%
Hospice	16.4%	4.6%	2.3%	33.4%
Physician Arrangements				
Independent physician association	4.6%	2.3%	1.7%	12.0%
Group practice	11.2%	3.3%	0.9%	12.2%
Physician/hospital organization	7.9%	3.1%	4.3%	3.5%
Management service organization	4.1%	3.5%	0.9%	3.0%
Medical foundation	1.9%	2.4%	0.3%	2.5%
Other	3.1%	0.8%	0.2%	2.2%
Insurance Products				
HMO	5.6%	4.4%	3.0%	21.2%
PPO	11.4%	5.7%	4.0%	24.5%
Indemnity/fee-for-service	8.4%	2.2%	0.7%	17.2%
Other	1.3%	0.6%	0.3%	2.2%

Note: Because hospitals could provide multiple responses, percentages do not add up to 100 percent.

(Tucci, Linda, "AHA Stats Verify Network Expansion," *Materials Management in Health Care*, Vol. 4, March 1, 1995, pp 80.)

(The 1994-1995 edition of AHA Hospital Statistics can be ordered by calling 800 AHA-2626.)

Though this is a logical response to market pressures, it is a wide swing from the ways in which hospitals have traditionally operated. Hospitals in metropolitan areas have structured themselves around inpatient services and utilization of specialists. The shifts to preventive care and strong dependence on primary care have been a change that has not only strategic but cultural implications.

Hospital administrators, their boards and medical staffs are striving to work together to build strategic alliances and/or formal partnerships. They may consider an urban hospital linking with rural hospitals to provide a referral linkage; they may form a Physician Hospital Organization (PHO); they may become the target of a large for-profit chain for purchase. In other words, their future is extremely uncertain. The nonvariable, however, is that the relationships, organization and governance must change to survive in today's market.

Some specific barriers to change faced by hospitals include:

- ***Legal and Other Restrictions.*** Public hospitals (numbering approximately 1,500) face unique barriers in the legal and political limitations imposed by state statutes, their community image, limited scope of powers, etc. These organizations are often unable to compete with nongovernmental entities. Following is an illustration:

  Public hospitals have a specific scope of legal authority that keeps city and county hospitals from engaging in nontraditional, health care-related activities. Some examples are durable medical equipment companies, commercial laundries, ownership in medical office buildings and the like. In Alabama, the retail florists challenged the hospitals' gift shops for selling flowers and thus engaging in commercial business. These restrictions are fraught with legal and political consequences.

  To compete successfully, many hospitals have chosen to restructure. This has often involved the sale of a hospital to a nongovernmental agency such as hospital chains. In other models, the public body retains ownership of the real estate and leases it back to a newly formed tax-exempt organization. These models require many assurances to the governmental agency regarding the issues of services, programs, uncompensated care, etc., and should include a deliberate and well-planned restructuring of the board of the corporation.

  The issues facing public hospitals often slow their progress in dealing with new linkages and offering new lines of business. Hospitals can remedy the structural issues, for the most part, but the change is often slow and the political fallout often continues well into the next generation.

- ***Issues Concerning Power.*** Whom has the power? This is one of the most significant issues facing a hospital and medical staff who are attempting to restructure their relationship and move forward together. It is also, unfortunately, one that is often not solved early in the venture and leads to its ultimate failure. Neither party can "take over" the other if they are truly going to partner. The issues surrounding power and money must be clear and expectations understood by all parties to the transaction.

- ***Image and Market Identity.*** In many communities, the hospital provides a strong economic base. The public has often come to see it as "their" hospital. This has been a goal of the marketing departments for years. To keep key stakeholders informed about changes and to continue their feeling of identity with the organization will be crucial to maintaining a market share. If the community does not feel the hospital and/or its medical staff continue to value their "personal" relationship, they will be less likely to remain loyal as options are presented to them from other organizations.

- ***Strategic Planning.*** We might regard this as "the choice between the devil and the deep blue sea ...." Strategic planning has traditionally been an orderly process based upon an assessment of the environment and logical extrapolations of what the future might hold. The current environment is chaotic and demands new thinking about planning. Hospitals have traditionally done long-term planning whereas physicians—their new partners— have traditionally planned for the short term. If one takes a moment to consider the differences in training between physicians and administrators and further looks at the subset of physician specialties, understanding this premise is not difficult.

Physicians are trained to assess and act. That is the very nature of the provision of patient care. If a third party required that a care giver test his plans against three distinct models before deciding a patient's course of treatment in a high risk situation, the results would be disastrous. We count on physicians to make fast, accurate assessments and to move forward.

The industry, in contrast, has traditionally afforded hospitals the luxury of scanning all aspects of the environment, building a series of scenarios, and testing them against models. Upon obtaining response from a variety of audiences, drafting and redrafting them, presenting them to boards, they then move forward toward application.

Neither approach will be entirely successful in today's market. Hospitals must speed up their planning approaches, continually test their assumptions, make decisive changes as appropriate, involve physicians in all aspects of planning, keep their eye on the ball and simplify their process.

Physicians, on the other hand, need to proactively insert themselves in planning, helping the hospital move forward more quickly and insisting that planning takes place *between* them—not by the physicians ratifying the hospital.

These changes will reorganize our planning process and allow us to learn to operate in this fast-paced environment. We will learn to take calculated risks, to make mistakes, to recognize them quickly, control the damage and continue to move forward.

- ***Bureaucratic Process.*** Academic medical centers are dilemmas in and of themselves. Approximately 6 percent (300) of the hospitals in the country are academic medical centers and yet they account for 20 percent of all inpatient admissions. They are a dominant economic, political and cultural force in the markets where they are found and beyond. They are also in trouble. With the decrease in reimbursement on multiple fronts, the move toward preventive health services and the market's dependence on primary care physicians, these centers (with their strong bureaucracies, their large specialty and research presence and the involvement of state and federal government) have more than a standard set of hurdles to jump.

They must reengineer to meet the demands of the market and, also, stay true to their mission. They must reinvent the relationships they have with government, universities, medical schools, etc., to allow innovation. Though this would be a difficult task, some consider the lack of skill and commitment by deans and department chairs to move quickly to a market-based system to be even more daunting. Cultural changes are always more painful, more difficult and slower than renegotiating contracts and legal arrangements.

The debate continues regarding whether the academic hospitals will rise to the occasion though the horizon is beginning to offer some hope.

- The UCLA Medical Center has become very aggressive in attempting to dominate its market. It has purchased the Santa Monica Hospital, developed a primary care network and created a strong referral service as part of its overall strategy for success and survival.

- The University of Wisconsin Hospital and Clinics, Madison, has worked with the Wisconsin legislature to create a public authority model that will move the day-to-day issues of the organization out of the hands of the state, thus allowing the medical center to pursue more innovative strategies. A recent joint venture with Blue Cross of Wisconsin and HMO Wisconsin has resulted in their own HMO product.

- Late last fall in Minneapolis, the University of Minnesota Health System and Fairview Riverside Medical Center (Fairview Health System) announced a merger that is receiving a good deal of attention. Competitors to the Fairview System are very interested in how the new arrangement will handle the State and Federal dollars that flow into the University.

- The State University of New York and academic medical centers in Pennsylvania, Florida and elsewhere also have considerable activity.

It is far too early to judge the success of these strategies. These undertakings are noble, however, as these medical centers attempt to survive by entering the market in new and untried ways.

■ ***Recruitment Challenges.*** Rural hospitals have their own special concerns. They are collaborating more strongly, forming networks and seeking to tie into larger centers for survival. They too face a wide range of political and cultural issues in this attempt. Coupled with the difficulty in recruiting primary care physicians to many of their locales, the efforts they are making in diversification, entering new service markets and recreating their structural arrangements are extremely challenging.

- **Competitive Alliances.** Recent news on the horizon cites the mergers between hospitals and insurance companies. Columbia/HCA will acquire most of Blue Cross/Blue Shield of Ohio and Aetna Life and Casualty is buying U.S. Health Care, Inc., a health maintenance organization based in Pennsylvania. Going forward, this market will have no shortage of partnering arrangements.

In examining their strategies for the future, hospitals must also look at protecting their bond ratings—this requires a strong alignment of financial incentives between physicians and hospitals. In 1994, Moody's Investors Service Inc., New York City, lowered seven California hospitals' debt rate resulting in increasing financing costs for these organizations. Their level of physician-hospital integration, in Moody's view, will determine the impact on credit quality. When hospitals make large capital investments in buying practices and setting up networks, this may adversely affect their credit. As a result, when hospitals set their integration strategies, they must also pay close attention to the impact on bond ratings, which could increase their net margins and lower their access to capital.

Hospitals have traditionally been the focal points for the health care industry and an economic stronghold in the community. The industry is now asking them to move from traditional roles, view themselves as a cost as opposed to a revenue center, partner with former competitors, behave collegially, reshape their governance structures, cut their costs, measure their outcomes, transform their cultures and "make it snappy." A tall order indeed!

Organizational Models to Allow Physicians and Hospitals to Partner

Terms

In this section, we will examine several physician/hospital partnership models. To fully understand the concepts, we must understand some terms. The list below is not exhaustive and does not include all definitions occurring in every area of the country or industry. Its purpose is to bring us to common terms with the assumptions made here.

(A comprehensive listing of terms and definitions can be found in *Managing Managed Care in the Medical Practice,* another title in the *PRACTICE SUCCESS!©* Series, also available through the American Medical Association.)

Clinical Integration. As defined by David Anderson, a partner at KPMG Peat Marwick, Chicago and Stephen Shortell, Ph.D., clinical integration is "the extent to which patient care is coordinated across settings and sites of care" to achieve the best results.

Group Practice Without Walls (GPWW). In a Group Practice Without Walls, physicians align to contract with managed care companies as a group. The key to the success of this plan is strong alignment and centralizing administrative functions while maintaining independent office locations. Legal and financial requirements for forming a GPWW vary by region. Physicians should carefully investigate them before deciding to form this type of entity.

Additionally, reduction of administrative costs and centralization of administrative functions often means the group must move or not retain staff in individual offices. They should thoroughly examine the political and financial consequences of these decisions. If the group is unwilling to reduce its administrative overhead, it will not maximize the benefit of this arrangement.

The Group Practice Without Walls is no longer a model in popular use around the country. It is an example of early integration efforts.

Health Maintenance Organization (HMO). HMOs function in a variety of ways, but all function in a federally regulated environment. The variances lie in the methods of delivering care. Many characteristics are common. They contract with a network of providers (physicians, hospitals and others) to deliver care to a defined population of enrollees. HMOs provide individual participants with "packaged" health care services in exchange for a fixed monthly premium "prepaid" health care. Like insurance companies, HMOs accept premiums in exchange for financing the cost of covered medical care. Like a health care delivery system, they arrange to provide care either directly or contractually. Contracts are set with a restricted set of providers and hospitals for a prearranged period. They hold down health care costs by transferring significant economic risk to providers and limiting the number of approved services.

Though they are continually changing, six models are commonly recognized as of this writing.

- ***Staff Model.*** Physicians are salaried employees, although the HMO may have outside contracts for some medical specialty or medical consultant services.

- ***Group Practice Model.*** This model revolves around a multi specialty group of independent physicians who provide services to contracted members. It may also permit physicians to see members of other HMOs or non-HMO patients. Physicians use this model in states that prohibit the employment of physicians by nonphysicians (the corporate practice of medicine).

- ***Network Model.*** The HMO contracts with several physicians or physician groups to provide services, securing a network to meet the demographic and geographic needs of the enrollee base. This network includes selected hospital and outpatient service sites.

- ***Independent Practice Association (IPA)-Type Model.*** This model uses (generally) multiple corporations formed by physicians who are each maintaining their practices. They participate in an Independent Practice Association to secure managed care business and provide a vehicle for accepting financial risk for members through capitated or discounted fees. This model provides good positioning for physicians to assume the responsibility for providing care to members in exchange for a fixed amount per member each month. The IPA spreads the risks throughout its members. It also offers a variety of physician compensation mechanisms. Generally, specialists are on a discounted fee-for-service basis and primary care physicians are on an individual capitated basis.

- *Direct Contract Model.* In this model, the HMO contracts directly with a panel of physicians, relying heavily on primary care physicians. These physicians act as care managers (or gatekeepers) for delivery of direct services and assumption of responsibility for making referrals to specialists. Each physician on the panel bargains independently with the HMO as an individual or through his or her small group practice.

  - *Specialty HMO Models.* In these models, the HMO is contracting in one area of medical specialty, such as orthopedics or obstetrics to provide prepaid coverage to its members. These models are often set on a discounted fee-for-service basis.

Independent Practice Association (IPA). An IPA is a corporation formed by physicians who maintain their independent practices but participate in the IPA to secure managed care business. IPAs accept financial risk for their members through the capitation or discounting of fees. The group is spread out geographically and is generally well positioned to provide a wide range of access for patients. The IPA providers (physicians) contract directly with the insurance company and, in many communities, directly with employers.

IPAs were originally formed to allow independent, community-based physicians a vehicle to compete with staff and group model HMOs. IPAs typically have a core of primary care physicians acting as gatekeepers who, besides providing primary care services to patients, manage all medical services and authorize all referrals to specialists. Experts disagree about the long term success of an IPA to compete effectively against staff and group model providers due to the inherent efficiencies in these other models.

Nevertheless, some markets (most notably California) are seeing strong growth and success through IPAs. Moody's Investors Service analysts have noted that physicians in California are "at the forefront of forming large physician groups and independent practice associations" that are able to negotiate capitated, risk-bearing managed care contracts. They are able to negotiate agreements with HMOs that hospitals have not been able to obtain. The physician groups are becoming overwhelming competitors who have consolidated their power effectively. ("Moody's Urges Caution," Jon Asplune, Copyright 1996, American Hospital Publishing, Inc.)

Today's marketplace has blurred the distinction between IPAs and PPOs, and they are becoming more integrated by providing some administrative services. Independent IPAs (not associated with any specific HMO), formed and controlled as a contracting vehicle by and for physicians, are becoming common.

Integrated Delivery System (IDS). This term has multiple definitions and is perhaps one of the most often discussed and least understood terms in the virtual lexicon that is emerging in the industry today. In its purest form, an IDS provides "seamless" care across a continuum through a variety of providers to include physicians, hospitals, insurance companies, HMOs, MSOs and other health care organizations. We can further define it as desegregation, blending, combining, consolidating, mixing and uniting health care services.

A key integrated delivery system strategy is to provide services along a spectrum of care to meet the full range of needs of the population it serves.

Management Service Organization (MSO). MSOs relieve the physicians of the administrative duties of running a practice while allowing them to retain ownership of their patient charts and records. The organization is set up by either physicians, a hospital, or an independent party. It furnishes services (such as facilities, staff, support services, administration of managed care contracts, etc.) to individual physicians, IPAs, PHOs, foundations (medical), medical groups, etc., on a fixed fee or percentage of gross revenue basis.

The MSO can have an exclusive contract with one professional corporation or a contract with more than one professional corporation. The physicians in the professional corporation can be independent contractors, employees or partners in the corporation. The physicians retain the patient charts typically (unless they are employees of the corporation) while the MSO purchases the tangible assets and leases them back to the physicians.

Most MSOs of not-for-profit hospitals are for-profit subsidiaries. Qualifying an MSO as not-for-profit can be difficult.

Other Weird Arrangement (OWA). On a lighter note, the Managed Care Answer Book, 1995, Panel Publishers, a division of Aspen Publishers, offers "Other Weird Arrangements" as a fall back acronym for arrangements that have yet to fit other accepted definitions.

Physician-Hospital Organization (PHO). A PHO is an organization structured traditionally with 50 percent control and ownership by physicians and 50 percent control and ownership by the hospital. PHOs are established to secure joint contracts with third party payers and often serve as an initial transitional model for the physicians and hospitals to learn to begin to work together.

The term PHO is also generically used to represent many different types of physician and hospital relationships and integration models. PHOs are often seen as transitional models in that they can be the first organizational step for a medical staff or group of independent physicians to learn to work together. Traditionally, they have had difficulty moving to a model where a single signature can commit the entire group.

Preferred Provider Organization (PPO). PPOs are networks comprising a panel of independent physicians with whom health insurance companies and health benefit plans contract for health care services at a discounted fee.

Some payers provide options for patients selecting to see physicians outside of the PPO. The patient can choose his or her provider at the time services are needed/provided. The first level of insurance coverage in which the provider is within the PPO network of providers, offers the highest coverage, typically 90 to 100 percent of covered services. The second level, for services provided outside of the PPO network, still provides benefits, but typically at a minimum of 20 percent lower than the In-Network benefit. Sometimes these are called Double Option plans.

This difference provides a financial incentive to the patient to utilize preferred providers, thus enabling the insurance company to demonstrate channeled (or directed) business to a provider in exchange for a discount. This channeling effect, in addition to utilization review, limited drug formulary, preadmission authorization and other mechanisms, also contributes to managed care discounts.

Primary Care Network (PCN). Primary Care Networks are seen as the centerpiece of providing care in today's environment. They generally include family practice and general internal medicine, often pediatrics and, in many markets, OB/GYN. This group of physicians is called upon to be the primary access point for the patients of the managed care organization, hospital or system with whom they affiliate. Physicians in these models serve in a care coordinator or gatekeeper role to provide the first line services for patients and determine an appropriate level of referral.

The physicians in the networks may be affiliated in a number of ways:

- part of a network or many networks contracted with by managed care organizations;

- members of an MSO or PHO who are obligating them to an agreed upon contract with a managed care organization or employer;

- fully employed physicians of a system, hospital or managed care organization;

- equity partners in a practice management arrangement.

Regardless of the structures from which they operate, these physicians are generally at risk for the overall performance of the network in the managed care contract. They have a difficult role to play in a fast changing system. Their jobs are fraught with political issues brought on by the environment, their specialist colleagues and other primary care providers who may or may not be a part of the network. They have the additional burden of having to serve as an interface between the patient and the managed care organization when certain levels of care are not authorized by the MCO. These primary care physicians are a major force in making today's system work as efficiently as possible.

Physician Organization (PO). Physician Organizations are models that are formed by and between groups of physicians. They take the same general shape and have the same goals as a PHO, but do not include the hospital as a partner. They vie for business with insurance companies and employers. They can subcontract work to one or more hospitals and can negotiate, en masse, for a preferred rate. Physician organizations require a fair amount of capital and may have an insufficient service offering in the long run to be sustainable as an independent organization.

Models

Physician–Hospital Organization (PHO). PHOs, which were virtually unheard of five years ago, are now common in many health care markets for a variety of reasons. They are often one of the first, and generally a transitional step, in the beginning of partnering between physicians and hospitals. They can coexist with Physician Organizations (PO), which may co-own the PHO but are generally formed as a single organization with shared governance between physicians and hospitals. The players in a PHO generally know each other and have worked together before, albeit in less of a partnership, and feel more in control than if they were contracting with an insurance company or other entity less familiar and often seen as less collegial. So, how are they faring, and should you join or start one?

Though many PHOs began to evolve over the past four years or so, the ones that are becoming contracting entities have seen their greatest strength come in the past two years. The first year can be an expensive, exhausting venture requiring a high level of meetings and decisions to be made. Though the process can be tedious, physicians need to be actively involved to ensure the final product will be one that meets their needs and the hospital's needs. Many physicians do not initially support the formation efforts of the PHO, and all parties are often reluctant to share information, decisions and power with the others. Payers are seldom entirely enthusiastic about contracting with a new entity that is struggling to get on its feet, so the startup can be quite discouraging for everyone. In its first year, most members do not feel the efforts have paid off, either in terms of making managed care contracting easier or more financially attractive. Nor do they feel they are responding with more speed than they could as an independent provider. If there are not visible improvements in volumes, payments or hassle reduction, it is difficult to keep the energy needed to continue the formation and operation of the PHO.

During the second year, the participants are more neutral than negative about the experience. They are beginning to make aggressive plans and see a difference in the general strength and organization of the PHO as a result of the work done in the first year.

They frequently still have not made significant inroads into managed care contracting. Yet, they are beginning to see how it can happen and becoming more confident about their strategy.

When PHOs enter their third year, they are once again often having to consider some reforms.

- If they have taken every provider who applies to the PHO, they may need to reduce the numbers and/or ratios of primary care to specialists. The current thinking among payers is the ratio should be 50-50 and many medical staffs are significantly overbalanced by specialists. These decisions begin to divide the medical staff and the selection criterion is always suspect, regardless of how it has been determined. It is during this time the PHO must make some difficult decisions. In addition to meeting the payers' needs for specialty/primary care ratios, the PHO must be careful about over-expanding the provider base in relationship to the volume of patients it can deliver. If the PHO patients are not a significant percentage of the PHO members' practices, the influence on practice styles and behavior will be difficult to influence. The vast majority of PHOs did not start with membership restrictions; now, two-thirds strongly consider that policy.

- During the third year, the data gathered on providers over the first two years begins to have some credibility. The dilemma now is what to do with the results? Is the organization going to make economically-based credentialing decisions? Is the criterion for membership strong enough, fair enough and administered equitably to stave off accusations and/or litigation regarding unfair treatment?

- PHO exclusivity is another issue becoming more prevalent. Can the physicians belong to other PHOs? How about other PHOs that contract with the same payers? Can the hospital compete with the PHO in payer contracting? The PHOs that are maturing are seeing these issues as new challenges to their solidarity and viability.

- Hospitals continue to provide more than half of the capital needed for the PHO, yet they maintain 50 percent or less of the governance structure. This financial inequity can potentially place the venture under regulatory scrutiny for Medicare Fraud and Abuse. These statutes prohibit the purchase of referrals and forbid private inurement to physicians. The capitalization of the PHO has associated regulatory, power and cultural issues and must be considered carefully in the initial and subsequent phases of development.

- Nearly one-third of the PHOs currently in operation are considering physician practice acquisition, and approximately 10 percent are now involved in this undertaking. This is a high risk strategy depending upon the market forces, the number of specialists, the competition within the marketplace, etc. Primary care practices, not specialists, are targets for acquisition. This creates tension, not only within the PHO, but moves back into the traditional medical staff of the hospital, since that is often the group from which the PHO membership originated.

- PHOs also offer management services, such as billing and collection, information systems, etc. This often makes the PHO more attractive, especially in its early stages. To be seen as added value to the physicians, management of these services must be pristine and well priced.

Determining Whether to Join a PHO

Asking the following questions will help you determine whether to join a PHO.

- **When was the PHO formed and why?** Insight into the motivations behind the PHO formation can be gained from the answer to this question. An organization formed as a protective, "circle the wagons" measure, whose philosophy remains unchanged, has questionable long term success.

- ***What services are provided?*** If management services are provided, what are they, who coordinates them and how well are they priced? Check with other PHO members who use the services to determine their value and if they have decreased their overhead. If they are perceived as an "add on" expense, the PHO's mind set may be simply repackaging the old ways of doing business. This philosophy will not bring success.

- ***Does the PHO have its own staff?*** Up to 50 percent of PHO budgets go to the personnel it takes to run them. Given that investment, it is important to know how much staff is on board, what is their function and level of performance and what is the experience/ background of the senior management or manager. To whom does the manager report? How often is his or her performance evaluated? What has been the track record? How approachable is the individual?

- ***What are the traditional and projected levels of investment of the parties?*** How is the organization capitalized? Does the collective wisdom think the current form of capitalization will hold in the future? Should it? What significance, if any, in the balance of power is based on the percentage of investment?

- ***What is the membership?*** Find out who belongs and what is the strategy for recruitment of more practitioners (and if they are specialists or primary care) and also how physicians can be removed from membership. These answers will help you look at the longer term strategies and some of the difficult decisions that may be required of the membership in the near future.

- ***What are the restrictions (if any) on belonging to multiple PHOs? On independently contracting with payers?*** Membership in the PHO is more than social or political. It can have major influence on how you are able to manage and expand your existing practice. Specialists, in particular, need to watch for restrictions. To deliver the volume of patients the specialists need, the market may demand that their services span many organizations.

- ***What current contracts or commitments does the PHO have with managed care organizations or directly with employers?*** Understandably, a new organization may have few or no current contracts. It should, however, have strategies for obtaining them and have a view of the market that can help them anticipate their level of success. Who will be responsible for obtaining these contracts, and what level of experience does that person have? How are the contracts reviewed, and who approves them for signature? These answers tell you a great deal about the level of involvement members can expect to have and allow you to determine, based on your personal viewpoint, if that is adequate for your needs.

- ***Who is at risk and how is that determined?*** Prior to signing anything, clearly understand the financial arrangements from setting fee schedules to determining risk pools. If the PHO has operated for a while and has some contracting experience, conduct a review of the success of that experience.

- ***How does the organization view itself three years down the road?*** This question is extremely difficult to answer in today's market and yet is an important one to ask. Although the environment is chaotic and accurate predictions are difficult to derive, the organization should have a vision or mission statement for its future. It should test against that goal to review its progress and verify its strategy. Does the PHO have a vision of where it wants to go and how to get there? Can it maintain its focus? Can it move quickly if it finds the market is dictating a change in strategy? These questions will give physicians good insight into the organization of the PHO and its commitment toward forward movement.

Though PHOs will probably evolve over time into other types of organizations, they are excellent starting points for beginning the difficult exercise of partnering. They provide physicians and hospitals with a vehicle for working together and for experimenting with other ways of thinking and conducting their mutual and their separate businesses. If the PHO is founded on protecting the group from the future, avoid it. Otherwise, the frustrations will be a distraction to exploring viable strategies to successfully meet the challenges in the changing marketplace.

Management/Medical Services Organizations

Management Services Organizations/Medical Services Organizations (MSOs) are other forms of integration physicians may find attractive. In the MSO field is a spectrum of assistance ranging from providing management services through the purchase and lease back of the tangible assets of the practice. These arrangements are favored because they can relieve the physician of the administrative burdens of the practice while allowing him or her to maintain full control over clinical decision making. (The physician maintains ownership of the patient charts and holds the HMO/PPO contracts.) MSOs also offer an integration approach for physicians in states that do not allow the corporate practice of medicine.

MSO arrangements require little capitalization when only management services are provided and the hard assets continue to belong to the physicians. Many of the services can be purchased from hospitals or other groups that own or sponsor the MSO. To take full advantage of the economies of scale in an MSO arrangement, the physician should work cooperatively with the MSO to reduce the overhead of the practice. For example, if the practice is to take advantage of the billing services offered by the MSO, they will need to eliminate the staff and systems that they currently employ and relinquish this responsibility to the management services organization. This concept is always easier to envision than to implement, especially when the smaller practices have tenured staff who may be unable to find other employment. The same can be said for the management and staffing of the office practice. Some staff members may be employed by the MSO, but one should not assume that no staff reductions will occur. Unless overhead can be reduced (and labor is a major expense), the MSO and the practice will not be successful in maximizing revenue and minimizing expense. A clear understanding of what services will be provided by the MSO, how they will be implemented and their impact on current staff should be reached before entering an MSO arrangement.

MSOs that purchase the tangible assets of a practice (and not all of them do) will require substantial capital. This capitalization often comes from the area hospital. Other arrangements for obtaining capital are made with private investors, the medical group or groups to be managed, HMOs or joint venture arrangements. Understanding the capitalization needs, the access to capital and the resulting tax implications (personally and corporately) of selling the practice is essential.

MSOs allow conveyance of the administration and management of the business. Physicians continue to maintain full decision making over the clinical aspects. While this is an attractive feature, one should not lose sight of the fact that physicians, not the MSO, continue to be at risk in HMO/PPO and other managed care contracts. The administration of the terms of the contract may be provided by the MSO, but the financial risk remains with the physicians.

Following are a number of reasons to enter an MSO arrangement:

- Access to capital through the sale of tangible assets;

- Access to information management systems whose capitalization will be spread through several groups instead of only your individual practice;

- Opportunity for smaller groups to have better access to claims management, professional administration, planning, marketing, joint purchasing, quality assurance systems, etc., that would be cost-prohibitive otherwise;

- Increased "clout" in dealing with managed care organizations;

- Clinical decision making remains clearly with the physicians.

Some of the potential drawbacks include:

- Loss of control over business decisions;

- The need to create a group consensus;

- The need to yield management to the MSO;

- A reduction and/or change in staff to realize economies of scale;

- The creation of a new culture due to combining with new groups/business partners in a way that has generally not been done in the past.

If you have decided to form or join an MSO, the following questions are worth your consideration:

- **Why?** Start with determining what you expect to gain individually and as a group. Test those expectations with your current and potential partners. An MSO can be analogous to an exclusive relationship—it is much easier to get into than to get out of.

- **How is the management to be selected?** An MSO's success depends largely on having strong, competent management. Even with the complexity of business decisions in the health care industry today, it is amazing how many practices are being managed by staff with no formal or experiential preparation to deal with the financial, legal and analytical issues facing all practices. If your current manager will be replaced in his or her role, are you ready to sever your relationship? Undertake the same analysis for each staff member. If members of the MSO are unwilling to downsize staff, cost savings will not occur. Thus, less money is available to capitalize information systems, site expansions, and other major expenditures.

- **How will you, as a practicing physician, interface with the MSO management?** This issue must be discussed with your colleagues and your potential business partner. The expectations of one another should be clear so all parties know what their accountabilities are and can be held to them. Leadership becomes more chaotic when there are no followers.

- **What are the tax implications of selling your tangible assets?** A Certified Public Accountant who is familiar with your practice and your own personal financial planner should analyze this issue. The answers to these questions will have major impact on how you structure the deal.

- **What services, specifically, will be provided by the MSO?** You will need to understand a number of things within your newly structured practice. For example, what is the policy on collections? If you have had a specific philosophy relating to that and your patient population has expectations built around it, will that philosophy be accommodated? What communications, if any, will be sent to the patient population, and who reviews them prior to mailing? Will there be a joint purchasing program, and if so, what criterion is being developed (and by whom) to determine the most effective purchasing partner(s)? Who is providing the marketing support, and how do they plan to market your practice? Who determines which contracts will be entered? Who is in charge of physician recruitment/succession planning and what is the agreed goal for mix of physicians and planning for retirement of those currently in the group who are nearing that juncture?

- **What is the approach being taken for the valuation of your practice?** Do you understand and agree with it?

- **If you decide to leave the practice, what are the penalties for such a decision?** Is there a difference in the "parting package" if you decide to leave the practice or if the

practice asks you to leave? Find out the terms of those two potentials. We often believe
we have settled into a location only to find that family emergencies and unexpected
events will necessitate our untimely change. The potential exists that you will breach
the MSO's contractual arrangements. Regardless of how remote the possibility seems,
get a sense of the ground rules in these circumstances.

- ***How will you measure the success of the MSO, and how often will you make a formal
review of the accomplishments of the organization?*** Rarely is the only measure of
success recorded on the financial reports. Look at the level of satisfaction you and your
colleagues have in working together, how the patients feel about their treatment, any
concerns about quality, staff turnover, contractual agreements, etc. All will have a role
in determining the success of an MSO arrangement.

In other words, notice what you are involved in now (both episodically and day-to-day)
and consider how you would like for the MSO to approach them in the future. Make
your needs known during the negotiation phase; do not wait until after the infrastructure
begins to take shape.

Finally, do not overlook or underestimate the time necessary to formulate the vision and
to consider the cultural implications of what you are assuming. These considerations are
far too often neglected by physicians as "soft stuff," yet can rouse the most discontent
over time. Unless all pull together, and have stated, discussed, documented and
periodically reviewed your direction, you will be pulled apart.

Primary Care Networks

Primary care networks, in their simplest form, consist of physicians in diverse geographic
locations providing patient care services. They can be loosely affiliated with one another
through contracts with a payer; they can be fully integrated into an integrated delivery system;
or they can be anywhere on the spectrum in between. When the term Primary Care Network
is tossed around, it refers to the primary care practices that are filling contractual arrangements
with an HMO or other organization. It may or may not be owned or providing a primary care
base for a hospital and/or system. Generally, they are owned.

A nonowned primary care network that contracts with a managed care organization has an
affiliation with that organization to fulfill certain contract terms, e.g., see the plan's patients,
provide an agreed-upon range of services, provide agreed-upon office hours, etc. The
physicians remain in their independent practices and are "networked" through this contractual
arrangement. No more, no less.

A primary care network is key to the success of any hospital, managed care organization or
system. The network provides the most common access for patients into the system. It can
serve as care coordinator for referrals to specialists and other services of the hospital, system
or managed care organization.

It is clear there is a shortage of primary care physicians in general and a severe shortage in nonmetropolitan areas. The current thinking is a ratio of 50/50 primary care to specialists best serves the patients and the payers. Most metropolitan areas have significantly more specialists than this new model will support, and fewer primary care physicians than they need.

Primary care physicians are being heavily courted by multiple organizations in an effort to control costs, provide access to services and establish linkages with their services or product. As a result, a number of options are available for these physicians/practices to consider.

Affiliation can take place in many forms. One of the primary strategies in Physician Hospital Organizations (PHOs) is to create a strong primary care base. The PHO becomes more attractive to managed care organizations and payers if they are located in the geographic areas of the population to be covered and will contract for necessary services. A network primary care physician serves in a "gatekeeper" or "care coordinator" role in establishing first line linkages with the patient, controlling referrals and assuming risk for the care provided to a population of covered lives.

A primary care network may be formed through a Management Services Organization's membership. These MSOs can represent the range of primary care physicians who belong to the MSO and often are in a stronger position to negotiate with payers than any freestanding individual practice. This is one of the MSO's advantages. Additionally, the MSO management should have strong skills in working with payers and employers to serve its members through a more appealing final contract.

Physicians may become salaried employees of a hospital or system. These systems acquire existing physician practices, employing the physicians to continue their practice. New physicians may be recruited to join existing practices, begin new practices and/or practice in urgent care settings depending upon the needs of the system and the payers contracting with the system.

Managed Care Organizations (either independent or part of a hospital/system) can contract with individual or group practices, for example, a Group Practice Without Walls (GPWW), to provide specific services for specific groups of patients. In this type of arrangement, the MCO is often only contracting for a portion of the total number of patients seen in the practice. The practice may serve as part of a primary care network for a number of MCOs or may have an exclusive arrangement. In the past, contractual arrangements were considered to be fairly short termed in nature. Traditionally, employers reviewed their health care plans annually and might or might not sign up with the same managed care organization multiple years in a row. New groups enrolled in the practice and previous groups left to begin a relationship with another group based on their insurance coverage. The group was left vulnerable to swings in patient volume and open to increased expense in the administrative functions.

Though the administrative issues are costly, the losses of continuity in patient care and the
turnover in doctor patient relationships are perhaps the most important prices paid by
physicians and patients alike. Primary care physicians, in the main, establish strong links with
their patients over time and have an excellent grasp on the physical and social issues of the
patient and his or her family structure. These are essential elements of managing care in the
most efficient manner possible. These multiple disruptions not only frustrate the patient and
the physician, but generally also have "real" costs associated with them. New relationships
must form with the physician having to catch up with what has been happening to the new
patient for prior years when they visited a different clinic or clinics.

In the quest to establish strong, long term relationships with primary care physicians, some
managed care organizations and systems are striving to create a long term partnership of ten
years or more. This presents the physician with an extended affiliation and a guarantee of
certain numbers of patients or reimbursement levels. Yet, the capitalization needs of the MCO
or System is reduced because the practice is not being purchased. As the move to preventive
care grows stronger, payers and employers will be more interested in affiliating with providers
of care who can demonstrate the long term effects of their wellness strategies. This can only
be done if the patients stay long enough in the network to track the outcomes.

Practice Acquisitions as Means of Forming Primary Care Networks

The interest in acquiring physician practices in the past five to ten years has moved along at
exponential rates. Many hospitals and other groups are acquiring practices and even more
physician groups are requesting to be acquired.

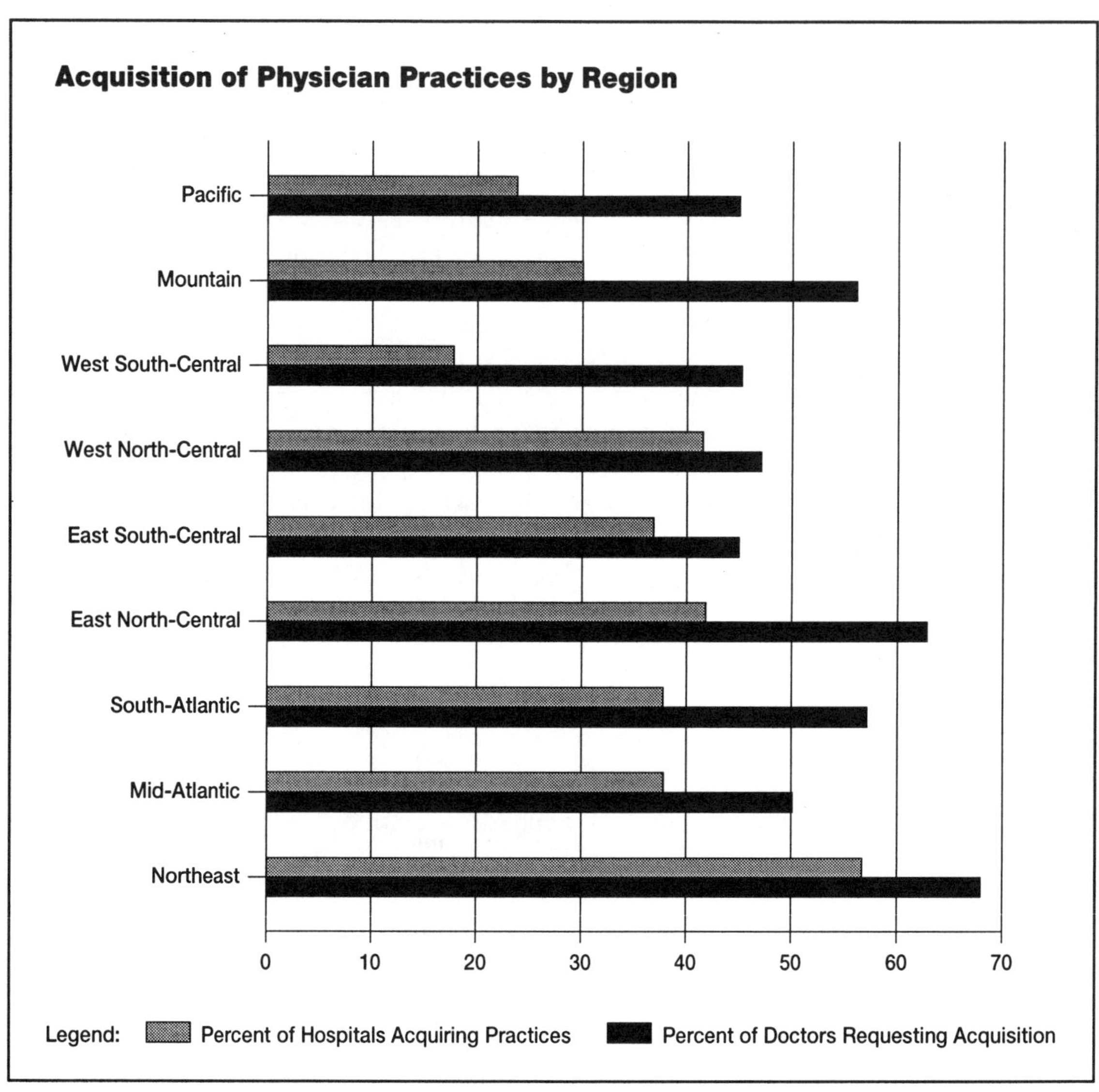

As the chart indicates, physicians and hospitals and other organized health care systems have major interest in practice acquisition. Systems (referring to hospitals, managed care organization, integrated delivery systems, etc.) are striving to provide networks to meet the demands of employers and payers. Physicians are looking for linkages to provide some measure of security and to ensure access to patients.

In some markets, the priority for building a primary care network has led to a panic mentality over purchasing physician practices. As the bidding wars heat up in highly competitive markets with strong managed care penetration, there is almost a feeding frenzy when it comes to practice acquisition. "Hi, I'm from XYZ Hospital have you been purchased yet?" Likewise, physicians have been deluged with offers and promises that seem almost too good to be true in a constrained market. They probably are!

A logical process can be used to sort out what is the best option for each party and to predict the success of the acquisition into the future. It takes some time and some planning yet is essential to the long term success of the venture.

The first step is to figure out what you are trying to do. This point seems almost too logical, but has not been taken all that seriously in the haste to acquire or be acquired.

What Do You, as a Physician, Want from the Network?

- **Is it access to capital?** If so, what capital is available and how can you obtain some of it? Having access to capital for expansion, upgrading and the like is often an advantage of being integrated into a system. It will be important to understand the capital planning process of the organization(s) who are considering purchasing your practice. Express your expectations or understandings early in the process. A look at what capital constraints they are anticipating is also of value.

- **Is it to ensure access to patients?** If so, what is the patient base of the suitor and what share will you see? What happens if/when those contracts no longer exist? If you are to be compensated on a productivity base in an area that has slow growth and an oversupply of physicians, to what is the organization willing to commit? Will you be asked to move into urgent care settings if this happens, and what voice will you have about those decisions after you become employed? Find out what the organization's track record is with regard to year-to-year retention of patient volume. Look at the patient mix. Ask if you will be able to/encouraged to see patients that are not members of the purchaser's managed care products or other networks.

  As you explore patient access, be sure your observation is through being part of a larger organization that can more successfully negotiate managed care contracts. Be certain you are not running afoul of Stark Laws I or II or federal fraud and abuse laws in your arrangements. Investing in the advice of an experienced health care attorney can be a wise decision.

- **Is it to have a sense of security?** If so, what can the potential buyer do to give this to you? All too often, the sense is that "someone has to keep us from the chaos." That will probably not be the case. Organizations can assist the physician to be more involved in patient care issues and less in the management of the practice, but the future and its many changes are still coming. Any organization you belong to (even if it is your original practice as a freestanding group) will need to flex and change in ways that may not always be to your liking.

- **Is it for financial gain as a result of the sale of your business?** If so, how is your business going to be valued? What are the tax implications to your group and to you personally as a result of the sale? Practice valuation will be discussed later; however, it is essential for you to understand how the purchase will be structured. Have your CPA/financial planner review the structure and advise you for your personal tax planning purposes.

- **_Is it to have a voice in the management of the network?_** Clarify what voice you will have and at what tables. Talk to others in the network to see if they feel they have a voice. Determine what a "voice" means? If the CEO of the group is a physician administrator, how does that person relate to the individual physicians in the group? Think about whether or not you are a consensus builder and whether you can live with decisions made by others on your behalf in the business. Look at your personal style to ascertain how much involvement you want to have, and then consider what time and energy commitments it will take to get you there. Also find out if the level of involvement you want is the level of involvement the purchaser is willing to extend to you. New networks have more than their fair share of nay sayers. Take a large sampling of the attitudes of others in the group, consider the maturity of the network, meet as many principals as you can in order to project how well you will work together in the long term.

- **_Is it to be part of a particular organization?_** If so, ask them what their plans are for the future. The organization you join today may be hardly recognizable five years from now. Although that is probably good, you should try to determine what the current plans are for growth and change. Multiple examples are available of clinics that were purchased by a hospital, the hospital integrated into a system, the system merged with another system and that merger moved forward to incorporate a large managed care plan. Overall, the system is probably much stronger than if it had not continued to respond to market pressures, but you may ultimately end up being a part of a system that does not resemble the one you joined. That, unfortunately, is difficult or impossible to control.

Generally, no single reason typifies why physicians consider selling their practices, but rather a combination of reasons often precipitated by recent market events. The more information you have from the network, its principals and members, the better off you will be in making your decision and in getting a feel for how well the system has thought through its acquisition strategies.

What does the buyer want from you? The old adage, "There is no such thing as a free lunch," has never been more true than in today's health care market. No longer are "great deals" out there as might have been obtainable even two years ago. Practice purchasers have become much more savvy and budgets are more constrained than when the shopping spree first began. Still, purchasers have limited experience, and they may be unable to articulate their performance expectations. It will be your responsibility to help them clarify their goals.

Clarifying questions:

- **_How do you plan to compensate physicians, during and after the initial purchase agreement?_** Will you be compensated on productivity? Does that include only gross professional charges? Is there a bonus incentive, and if so, is it based on the performance of your clinic, the network, the system as a whole or a combination? Find out how often the incentive bonus has been paid since the network was formed. Will your compensation be linked to the expenses of supporting you, and if so, what variable expenses can you influence?

- ***How are compensation plans being determined?*** As compensation plans change ("from time to time" as many contracts note), who develops them? What parameters are set by the system and what decisions are left in the hands of physicians? What, if any, payment can you expect for administrative work, board attendance, meeting participation and simular responsibilities? What are the base measures for "full time" work? What are the associated benefits? How often is "from time to time?" Is there a notice period? Will you be protected in some way from precipitous drops in compensation?

Other financial issues that must be addressed concern outside income from independent medical examinations for insurance companies, salaries for being on the boards or serving as medical director for outside organizations, etc. Those issues should be thoroughly discussed, and the contract should reflect the outcome of those discussions. Many physicians derive significant incomes from these arrangements, some of which require the use of office space and staff. If the office is owned by the purchaser and the staff is employed by the purchaser, what happens to the income derived. What are the billing arrangements that need to be made?

- ***What benefits are available?*** Know what the allowances are for CME (both in time and dollars), cellular telephones, professional association dues, subscriptions, long and short term disability, life insurance, tax-sheltered annuities, health and dental insurance, paid time off, holidays, and other parts of the package being proposed. If you are to work in an emergency room or urgent care facility, will there be additional pay for excess hours, holiday coverage, etc. Find out how many hours you need to work to obtain full time benefits and what benefits are available to you if you decide not to work full time.

- ***Who is going to manage this network and what experience do they have with clinics?*** One mistake made by hospitals purchasing clinics is to think the hospital administrators can manage the clinic as simply as another line of business. This is a dangerous assumption. Physicians often remind hospitals that clinics are not small outpatient units based away from the hospital. They are a different line of business and will require management with clinical expertise in order to maximize revenues and minimize expenses. It is often tempting, when purchasing clinics, to have staff serve in both hospital and clinic settings. Help the purchaser to resist this temptation. Be sure the management structure is of sufficient size and experience to ensure the support you are anticipating.

- ***What happens to my current support staff?*** For some physicians, this is a "deal breaker." The current staff is often left in tact and brought into the new organization "whole." They are given credit for vesting schedules and previous experience. Illness leave and vacation days accrued are either paid out or transferred. Good network managers will not pay clinical staff at hospital rates since this is not market-competitive.

Do not assume you have appropriate staffing levels or skill levels in your clinic to meet the new market demands. The purchaser will want or need to evaluate this over time and may make decisions you would not have made if this were still your own business. Keep in mind, deferring management decisions is one reason why you allowed your practice to be purchased. Work with the managers to move forward in efficiently and humanely. It is extremely frustrating for all concerned when physicians take an advocacy role between their former staff and their new management. The cooperation component is difficult yet a determinant in making the system work for everyone.

- ***What are the plans for network growth and mix of physicians?*** On what data was this decision based? As much as anything, this question helps the purchaser to look at the strategies they are using to expand their network. Does the population support the current plan? What physician specialties will make up the network and to what extent? What about your traditional referral base — are there plans to continue to use this group or must your referrals go elsewhere? Does the primary care network plan to employ any specialists or are they contracting with this group to meet the needs of the patients? How will the selection process take place?

- ***What are the work expectations?*** If there are base productivity levels and expectations the purchaser will have of you as a physician, these need to be articulated and clearly understood. How many patient contact hours per week in the clinic are expected for full time? How do call shifts figure in? Are you expected to cover urgent care clinics, provide evening hours, assist in the emergency room, provide hospital coverage for the patients under your care and/or the care of others? What are the short and long term disability benefits if you should become sick, pregnant or injured? Are there expectations that you serve on a certain number of hospital or clinic committees? What do they expect from you in the area of quality assurance initiatives?

- ***Is there an expectation this network will "break even" and what does that mean?*** This can be tricky. It will take time, especially if practice acquisition activity is brisk, to determine a common fee schedule, appropriate staffing levels, assure coding compliance, etc., that will impact the financial performance of the group. "Break even" is also influenced by the ability of the network to secure new business and retain its current volumes. The financial projections must necessarily consider the costs of recruitment, equipment, etc., and will have strong cash requirements. The network must be given time to meet performance targets. Current thinking is that the network can expect to lose from $18,000 to $25,000 per physician annually and more if the network is continuing strong growth. It is essential to take this information in concert with the other benefits to the system such as the sale of managed care plans, referrals to the tertiary centers and the like. In the practice acquisition game, the theory of spending money to make money is alive and well. Network administrators should have a strong and realistic understanding of this inevitable outcome. They should not prematurely pressure the network to perform to the same general expectations they have held for hospitals. However, administrators should work with physicians who are performing outside the norm. Financial performance "does count." It is to say the system needs to take a long view regarding this strategy and be able to fund the enormous startup financial needs fully.

- **What are the plans for integrating the different parts of this network?** If the network comprises geographically disparate clinics, will you/should you know your colleagues and will there be a plan to accomplish this? If hospitals are in the system, how will the network interact with them and what are the expectations? The same question applies if there are associated health plans.

- **What data is collected about physicians, how is it used and what is your access to it?** It is always important to know what information is being collected for credentialing and financial performance purposes. Will the network share with you how your performance is in comparison to your colleagues? If your style of practice is more expensive than the others, what do they plan to do with the information and how will you be expected to respond? How is this data shared with the system's health plan? Is it shared with other health plans? How often can you expect a "status report" on your individual performance and that of your work unit?

- **What happens in the event you want out or the system wants you to leave?** Be sure you fully consider any noncompete clauses in your contract to ascertain if they are reasonable and enforceable. What happens to the purchase pay out if you leave before the term of your agreement? Will they pay you for any leave you may have accrued? Are there penalties for withdrawing early from any of the benefit plans? Having this information available and understood in case you want or need to leave the organization will prevent many misunderstandings in the future if you should sever your relationship under amiable or less than desirable terms.

Systems purchase practices and employ physicians for many good reasons, and physicians have many good reasons for choosing to become employees. The key to determining whether this is an appropriate choice for you comes in understanding the terms of the deal on the front end and, as possible, eventually before making a commitment. If the system and you are dissatisfied with one another and you have no remedies at your disposal, the opportunity to enjoy your practice and your affiliation is extremely limited.

Physician Employment Models

(The section of this book dealing with primary care networks addressed a number of considerations when contemplating full employment by a hospital, HMO or Integrated Delivery System. The purpose of this section is to describe the various models operating in the market today. These sections are not exclusive of the other.)

The concept of physician employment models is straightforward. In states where there are no regulations against the corporate practice of medicine, hospitals or foundations can directly employ physicians instead of forming a separate professional services corporation. These employment contracts, when done well, explain the compensation arrangements (a salary guarantee is generally available for the first year or two), the benefits, the description of expectations, noncompete clauses, termination clauses and, as applicable, signing bonuses, loan repayments, relocation expenses, etc. The contracts are fairly standard and should be reviewed by the physician's attorney prior to signing.

A second model is the equity model, which is generally a for-profit structure that employs physicians. Funding can come directly from the physicians who own, operate and govern the practice. Hospitals or systems may contribute an equity investment if they think the entity has significant strategic importance. Then, the hospital/system would be an investor or part owner in the practice. In that these are for-profit structures, access to capital may be an issue for the group. They are not eligible for any tax-exempt funding. On the other hand, tax-exempt funding can carry several restrictions with it that make it difficult to flex quickly in today's market. In these physician-owned equity models, the physicians may contract for hospital beds or purchase a hospital.

Professional Practice Management (PPM) companies also offer equity purchase arrangements with physicians. In those structures, part of the revenue flows back to physicians for providing the services and a portion flows to the PPM. Physicians own the PPM (often as part of the financial package for selling their practice). Because the physicians benefit from the revenue stream in two ways, they have extra incentives to reduce their overhead and maximize their revenues. Some of these models have gone public and more are considering that option.

Here is how it works: The PPM purchases the physician practice in exchange for stock in the PPM and a negotiated cash amount; the physician contracts with the PPM for management services. Since the physician is an equity partner in the PPM, he or she receives benefits from the success of the PPM beyond the payment received for providing patient services. These PPMs are relatively new and have not had adequate time to test for long term success. Many physicians would rather work for a physician-owned entity as opposed to a hospital, system or managed care organization. The physicians may be able to bargain with hospitals and payers in their particular market for more attractive managed care contracts. The agenda of the PPM and the practice can be kept "clean" since physicians have no ties to any particular hospital or system. They can negotiate and refer patients to whatever groups provide the highest quality of care in the most efficient manner.

Whether this model will be popular in the community (they are primarily in California and the southern states now) should be well tested before entering into such an arrangement. Obviously, if the physician stands to gain from the practice and the PPM, they are also accepting risk depending upon the success of both.

The real key to physician employment models lies in being able to make them work. You can structure almost anything, but it takes much more than contracts, cash and lawyers to establish a long term, satisfactory partnership.

Physician–Physician Relationships

Introduction

This section will concentrate on physician to physician relationships and explore some organizations and structures that enable physicians to form networks independent of payers, hospitals, and systems.

To maximize the understanding of the physician to physician relationships, some background information is in order.

The Only Constancy is Change

The journals are full of information about primary care physicians, their new roles, the shortage of practitioners, maldistribution, etc. Indeed, the role the payers, and following them, the patients, expect primary care physicians to play has changed over the past five years. So has the role of the specialist.

As partnerships form in the health care markets of this country, not losing sight of the role and culture changes affecting physicians in all segments of the industry is essential.

Primary care physicians are being pushed into problem solving roles within the newly emerging markets. They are not only required to take care of patients with quality and cost-effectively, but also to manage the economics and advocacy issues of patients and payers. Most physicians did not train for this role and, even more, never wanted it in the first place. Only 29 percent of U.S. physicians are considered primary care physicians. Great Britain boasts 72 percent while Canada and Europe have 50 percent. The current thinking generally considers an ideal balance between primary care and specialists to be a 50/50 ratio, yet only 14 percent of U.S. medical school graduates were planning to enter the primary care field in 1992. Many primary care physicians are also in the population in the later stages of their careers and are looking forward to retirement. Adding to this dilemma is the maldistribution of primary care physicians in the rural parts of our country and the increasing dissatisfaction with the problems being thrust at this segment of the physician population. (These issues have little to do with practicing medicine and a lot to do with managing the business of health care). Residency programs are beginning to provide some direction and education concerning business and managed care issues. However the efforts may be too little too late.

Though primary care physicians are currently being cast in a role of managing access, the final evolution will be to manage care. They will be concentrating on improving the health care of individuals and populations, not limiting access or playing "gatekeeper" for a managed care organization. Their role today is a transitional one. This role will potentially damage the relationships between primary care providers and their specialist colleagues and possibly primary care physicians and patients who feel they are being under served. The key is to manage the transition well and to look to the outcomes of care over the long term.

Specialists have also seen market forces change their practices dramatically in the last five years. Many patients, due to their insurance coverage, cannot refer themselves for care to a specialist without first seeing a primary care physician. The populations who would, in the past, call an orthopedist with a sore joint, or set an appointment with a gastroenterologist when having a GI problem can no longer access the highest levels of their insurance companies if they continue this practice. This has led to a situation where the specialists have had to team with primary care in ways never before thought of and in ways previously untried. Further, many physicians who formerly had a "referral only" practice in areas such as internal medicine subspecialties are now devoting part of their practices to general primary care to obtain patient access and keep their practice volumes at reasonable levels.

Added into the fray are hospitals who are carving market nooks in services that were previously performed in the physician's office. Womens' health care centers, sports medicine, cardiac rehabilitation and, most obviously, urgent care are impinging on areas that were previously part of the physician's exclusive practice. These shifts are also taking patients and revenues out of the office settings. Hospitals, on the other hand, are concerned about physicians who have their own radiology departments and laboratories. The physicians once would have referred all or most of this business to the hospital.

Everyone is changing roles, participating in new-to-them service ventures, concerned about access, quality and cost, and merging cultures. More often than not, they are finding themselves in a financial and political morass.

Meanwhile, "back at the ranch," patients are demanding faster, convenient service; more voice in health care decisions; lower costs; increased choice and fewer hassles. In times past, patients were more compliant and more trusting in the medical profession. They did not demand or expect technology or pharmaceuticals to help them out of every situation. They even accepted death as inevitable. Patients partnered with their physicians in a trusting, therapeutic relationship that has been dramatically redefined over the last decade.

Enter the payer to the scene. The payer wants lower costs, happier customers, more business, greater access, physician and patient compliance, network participation, risk sharing and increasing involvement in clinical practice to accomplish these goals.

Further, the market is segmenting into employer coalitions, primary care networks, specialty networks, physician/hospital networks, for-profit networks and the like. The term "unstable atmosphere" no longer is reserved exclusively for meteorologists. It applies to health care, as well.

To determine the best relationship(s) a physician can have with the health care industry, looking at what is the underpinning of a successful alliance, how the marketplace evolves and what specific options are available today is important.

Underpinnings of a Successful Alliance

Evidence shows that many partnerships fail before really getting started. Since they are disruptive to the day-to-day business of providing care to patients, partners have a keen sense of urgency to "get the deal done quickly." (Green, J. "The Cost of Hospital Mergers," *Modern Healthcare*, February 3, 1992, p. 36.) Building partnerships is both tactical and strategic and will require a good deal of time, energy and money to be successful. Underestimating the resources necessary to change the face of the practice of medicine as known today is extremely shortsighted and will ultimately lead to failure.

As physicians review their options, they must come together around a sound business purpose that can provide what the market wants to buy. As "a rule of thumb," consider what someone will write a check for and provide that. Another truism is to decide what can put you out of business and become that.

Whatever the business reasons for forming groups or networks, you must participate with people/organizations you can trust. Eventually you will need to risk with a partner or partners, but do not move too quickly. Take time to consider the short- and long-range issues around being able to work through problems involving politics, money, power, control, etc. You do not have to be of like mind, but you do have to believe in the integrity of the other party to have a chance to succeed. You can read the books, go to the seminars, talk with your colleagues, get your MBA, "surf the Internet," and more, but at some point, you will be forced to make choices about how you are going to interact with the health care environment. Steps can and should be incremental, tested and, if necessary, changed before taking the next step. The first step requires courage and an honest evaluation of the results. It also requires the ability to recognize mistakes, reconsider and move on.

In its simplest form, the health care industry is learning to communicate and cooperate with former competitors. To determine the mission of the organizational structure and the core values surrounding it will be crucial to developing trust and accomplishing common goals. To overlook the communication and common vision needs is a risky strategy that has proven time and again to be the demise of well-intended groups lacking a commitment to common outcomes.

To determine what you are looking for, you must first look at what business you are in. In the global sense, it is generally improving or preserving the health of a given population and community. Try to be more narrow in your approach. Determine your core values.

The forming group needs some commonalities among its members. Practice styles, age, demographics, personalities, cultures, business goals and similar issues should be well explored. Look at your current colleagues as potential partners. Do you want to practice like them? Would you want them taking care of your patients? Would you be pleased to be named as a part of their group? How do they treat the clinic or hospital staff members? How do they treat you?

A physician leader who can move a group toward a consensus, is not conflict-averse and has a strong business sense is a key success factor. Physicians want and need physicians to lead the effort—not alone, perhaps, but in a key decision-making role. Physicians generally prefer to follow the lead of other physicians; further, the very nature of the business requires it.

Physicians must be aware of their competitors, including not only hospitals and payers, but other physicians who are competing in the same arena. A strong sense of survival is needed focusing on accomplishing the goals. An equally strong ability to make organizational changes in both the short and long term is necessary. Physicians see themselves as collegial. This is changing as the concerns about diminishing access to patients and payments in a constrained market become more defined.

The historical mistrust between hospitals and physicians is not new and will not change quickly. Further, as the market becomes more constrained and the need to work together as a team becomes more critical, skepticism by and among physicians can irreparably damage the newly forming alliance. A reduction in levels of trust should strongly signal the time to begin to talk about the issues—the real issues—as a partnership and begin to resolve and/or redirect the efforts. Staying engaged requires stamina and self-discipline when the organizational goals seem impossible to attain.

Physicians, largely, are accustomed to practicing on their own or in small groups. They are use to questioning business decisions and maintaining control. When organizational expectations for revenue and patients are not met, often the physicians pull back and lose interest in managing their day-to-day business. This is when trust in the partnership begins to fade. This is also the time to openly reassess and/or reaffirm the original goals that brought the groups to consider partnership.

Physicians have a key stake in both the short and long term economics. They must insist on being part of each decision and make certain they understand the business risks being considered. Especially in a capitated environment, there are major misalignments of incentives. For example, the hospital wants to fill its beds and physicians are operating under a per member per month payment system. The process for discussing and coming to agreement on how these opposing issues are to be handled calls for forthright discussion, compromise and clear understanding of the agreements reached. The economic issues are often cited as reasons ventures fail. In reality, it is not only the money, but the disillusionment with one another that makes the alliance unworkable. To identify the financial benefits each party expects while realistically evaluating the cost of the transaction and productivity issues is not an option. It is essential. Glossing over this step or not understanding it fully will result in a dismal outcome, no matter whom the partners are.

Know your market. It is different from what it was yesterday. Do not underestimate the rapidity of change. Build an organization that is constantly surveying the horizon and building contingency plans to deal with a variety of scenarios.

To review:

- Plan to devote the resources (including your time) necessary to research, form and develop the partnership no matter with whom you ultimately align;

- Determine your business purpose, articulate it and build the consensus around it;

- Be willing to assess your progress and make changes honestly as indicated;

- Become skilled at communication;

- Know your core values;

- Be intentional about deciding what business you are in;

- Look at your potential partners and determine compatibility;

- Select and support a physician leader;

- Be aware of your competitors;

- Assess and reassess trust levels;

- Continually be aware of control needs/wants;

- Understand clearly the economic issues, expectations and contingencies to address differences;

- Know your market;

- Keep your eye on the ball. . . .

Market Evolution

In spite of the chaos, you can predict the evolution of the market by considering some basic factors. In the Minneapolis market, a resounding wake up call came in 1993 when a consortium of twenty-four businesses issued a Request for Proposal for provision of services to their employees. Likewise, Chicago, New York and other parts of the country are seeing leverage applied by large single employers, employer coalitions and labor unions.

Also in 1993, legislative moves in New Jersey and New York had substantial impact on the organization and delivery of health services virtually overnight. Deregulation of the environment has resulted in competitive discounting strategies that had previously been illegal.

Industry analysts are keeping an eye on the Medicare and Medicaid programs and the various managed care strategies under development to access that huge population. A highly attractive managed care product to Medicare and Medicaid recipients will dramatically alter the landscape.

Other factors that suggest imminent change are the coalescing of physicians. Either through specialty organizations, IPAs, Group Practices Without Walls, primary care networks, or coalitions of many shapes and sizes, the coming together of physicians is a signal the market is on the brink of major change. Organizational structures have substantial influence over delivery of goods and services to the market. Operating in large blocks gives significant leverage to those who have organized.

The market is a composite of supply and demand. For massive change to occur requires a nucleus of physicians and other providers to conform. In other words, rural areas with few physicians do not have huge managed care penetration. They are, however, often key to the referral strategy of any number of networks. If you are in a rural setting, however, do not get too comfortable just yet. You are not immune to aggressive outreach programs from larger facilities within a reasonable drive of your locale, or to the increasing penetration of managed care organizations. Say, for example, a large national employer is in your community, such as a meat packing plant. The national organization could strike a deal with a physician network in a nearby town to provide for the health care needs of its employees. Think about the base of business you could lose through this move. Actions in Washington, D.C. will not change the health care scene as quickly as the employers who are attempting to protect their profits through a reduction in health care costs.

Physicians who think they can band together and keep managed care out are not realistic in markets where there are many physicians. The band will be broken by legislation and/or employers, if not by other physicians entering competitive arrangements. Swimming against the tide in a market that has the demographics to support competition is tiring and ultimately does not take you anywhere.

APM, Inc., a New York City firm and University Hospital Consortium, Oakbrook, Illinois, has done an excellent job of staging market evolution. Their findings were published by American Hospital Publishing, Inc., 1995, in an article written by Kevin Lumsdon, "How markets evolve... ," Volume 69, Hospitals and Health Networks, March 5, 1995, page 48. The study is well known and quite detailed. It can be accessed by contacting Debbie Dodge at APM, (312) 214-8683.

The article primarily works on the premise that "when you have seen one health care market, you have seen one market." Unstructured markets are those with little managed care, few hospital consolidations and few large physician groups. They continue to fill hospital beds (which are in oversupply) and are overused when compared with managed care markets. They operate on fee-for-service or discounted fee-for-service arrangements. Though they have not seen the changes of other markets, those changes are coming.

The second stage involves the beginning of hospital consolidations, early attempts of insurers beginning to partner with providers, organization of physician groups and deep discounts in inpatient care.

Consolidation heralds the beginning of stage three in which there is heavy managed care penetration, some capitation (especially in primary care), accelerated movement into groups (again, especially in primary care), specialists begin group formation, overcapacity begins to decrease and providers and insurers move to align incentives.

Managed competition is perhaps the most mature stage we have witnessed to date. Characteristics include strong alignment between providers and insurers, specialists see a sharp drop in fees, networks are utilized to provide a full continuum of care, HMO penetration exceeds 50 percent, fee-for-service payment is extremely limited and employer coalitions form to purchase health care services. Examples of this type of market are evident in Southern California (San Diego and Los Angeles) and Minneapolis/St. Paul, Minnesota.

The fifth stage will include networks with market share forming true partnerships with insurers, integrated systems manage care for patient populations, and providers begin to focus more sharply on their unique strengths. Pockets of this stage are beginning to emerge. The highest hurdle to clear is the partnership of providers and insurers the alignment of incentives in these long standing competitors.

As you look at your market, you can begin to assess what stage you are in and, using this staging as a guideline, where you might be headed. The following questions may help you with this analysis:

1) Have changes occurred in the way physicians are organized over the past 12 to 18 months? If so, what is happening? Are primary care physicians and/or specialists coalescing? Are they directly contracting with insurers or employers?

2)   Are employers forming coalitions to negotiate the price of providing health care for their employees?

3)   Are hospital beds in oversupply? Are hospitals attempting to consolidate with one another or with physicians? Are the hospitals purchasing physician practices?

4)   What is the state of "for-profit" management companies in the region? What is their vision for the market?

5)   Do you have employers in your community who may be part of a larger organization (perhaps not locally based) who are considering widespread changes on the corporate level that may affect your patient population?

6)   What is happening in contiguous regions to your community, in the closest metropolitan area?

7)   Is your referral base secure?

8)   What are you hearing from your local medical societies and the American Medical Association?

9)   What do the local physician leaders consider to be the most likely changes?

10)   How well positioned are you and your practice for change?

Change is happening rapidly. You must constantly monitor your environment and make informed decisions based on what you are seeing, learning and feeling. You are best able to monitor subtle change in your practice and community. Often, the subtle changes will herald the massive changes of the future.

You will also need to scan on a national level since the change of today is not respectful of geographical boundaries. Be prepared. Trying to keep up with the latest merger is somewhat like tracking the emerging governments of Europe. For example,

> Columbia/HCA Healthcare Corporation based in Nashville exchanged hospitals in West Valley City, Utah; Layton, Utah; and Milton, Florida with Paracelsus Healthcare Corporation for hospitals in Ormand Beach, Florida; Halstead, Kansas; and Jefferson, Louisiana.

> Tenet Healthcare Corporation, Santa Monica, California, has signed a definite agreement to acquire a hospital in Florida. This will expand their South Florida Health System network that owns 46 facilities including acute care hospitals, psychiatric and skilled-nursing facilities and out-patient-surgery centers.

Blue Cross of California has converted to for-profit status by merging with its for-profit subsidiary, WellPoint Health Networks, Inc. WellPoint is one of the nation's largest HMOs, with four million members as of First Quarter, 1996. Blue Cross will bring another 310,000 members to the deal.

In August 1996, Pacificare Health Systems, Inc., proposed a $2.1 billion acquisition of FHP International. If this deal is approved, it would result in the creation of the nation's fifth-largest health insurance company with four million subscribers.

These changes—whether they involve physician practices, hospitals or managed care networks will influence the environment and are worth watching for both signs of success and signs of failure. Many "free lessons" are out there but with no easy answers. You must stay informed to make your best choices.

The clues are there. The markets are changing daily. In a planned manner, you need to constantly, consistently and reassess your particular market and the strategies you are using to gain a competitive edge.

Options, Alternatives, Opportunities, Choices

Today's physicians are faced with having to make change. The status quo is no longer working and the market is moving at warp speed. Physicians are faced with choices that involve not only their personal needs, but the needs of their families, associates, the community and the system overall. They are called upon to employ new skills and perspectives. This is a difficult time.

More than anytime in history, physicians are reexamining their choice to pursue the practice of medicine in general, or their particular specialty or employment structure. Many are opting to move into careers that have previously been sideline interests such as teaching, writing, consulting, research, etc. They are finding sorting out the myriad of options to be extremely difficult.

If you are seriously thinking about changing careers, find a mentor (preferably another physician) who can add some objectivity to your thinking. Select your mentor carefully. He or she may or may not be a personal friend. For the best outcome, select someone who seems able to view you objectively. You will need to identify carefully why you are dissatisfied. Sometimes it is something that can be remedied (like a poor choice of associates); sometimes it will require change of specialty or career paths. Analyze the problem and gather data on possible choices. From that step you will be able realistically to look at your options and develop a plan of implementation. Having an "outside mentor" is essential to help you through this most difficult time if you are to consider the range of possibilities and the potential impact on your personal and financial goals.

This section will assume the physician plans to stay in medicine. It will examine some vehicles currently in use that can transform practice patterns and provide new linkages with new partners. One should keep in mind that new strategies are being introduced almost daily, and variations on a theme are plentiful. Many factors will influence the structure chosen, i.e., personal style, professional goals and market forces. Each vehicle described is presented in its current general template. Being able to take the best of each and adapt it to your situation will be key to your long term success and satisfaction.

The Solo Practitioner—an Endangered Species?

Today, 33.4 percent of physicians providing direct patient care are practicing in groups of three or more, compared with 18 percent in 1969. A recently reported study finds that physicians in groups of three or more feel they have less restriction on their autonomy, are more likely to be board certified, participate in Health Maintenance Organizations and generally have somewhat higher incomes than their colleagues in practices of one or two (34 percent). Further, 32.6 percent practice in other patient care settings, such as hospital employment or temporary employment arrangements. (Volume 3, *Presidents & Prime Ministers*, May 1, 1994, page 44, Douglas Hurd.)

As demonstrated by the severe shortage of physicians in rural areas, it is becoming more difficult to practice alone. Solo physicians and those in extremely small groups are finding they do not have the political or financial "clout" to deal with managed care organizations and the plethora of increasing regulations. Further, they generally do not have business managers with the experience to help them through this quagmire. They are no longer able to have successful practices simply by seeing patients and sending out statements. They are inundated with regulations regarding everything from how their laboratory is set up to coding compliance issues. The office is no longer a "personal business" but rather a component of a larger system that is reeling out of control. The ability to recruit associates in the practice of medicine to smaller groups and the need to enhance the business acumen of managers has led these physicians to link with other groups to maintain their financial viability. It has also led to exceedingly higher levels of frustration, anger and discouragement among the work force in the health care industry.

It has been suggested that due to the lack of managed care penetration in rural areas, physicians may find it easier to practice in these locations. As often happens, this suggestion has two sides to it. New residents coming out of school are often not interested in the solo practice opportunity. Being alone or with one or two partners, often far away from specialists and high technology, having to take call every night, etc., holds little interest. Further, the physician often has a spouse looking for employment opportunities that may not be present in smaller communities. In addition, though many employers have not moved to managed care yet, the Medicare population in these areas is often disproportionate, and thus the reimbursement levels are less than optimal.

Physician recruiters will attest to the fact that recruiting for a small group or solo practice is almost an impossible task. The physicians today are seeking more safety in numbers and have different lifestyle expectations than those entering practice thirty years ago. To find a quality associate to join a small practice takes magic; to find a physician who wants to buy the practice upon the retirement of the current physician is nearly impossible.

The day of the solo practitioner is quickly drawing to a close. Communities that will no longer have a physician, once the current doctor retires, will suffer both in personal and economic terms.

Group Practice Formation

To review, physicians are joining groups for the following reasons:

- Increased negotiating power with managed care organizations;

- Increased ability to recruit associates;

- Relief from administrative hassles including personnel issues;

- Access to capital;

- Access to professional business management;

- Better hours and call coverage arrangements;

- Overhead economies of scale (e.g., purchasing arrangements, staffing, billing, collection, etc.);

- Increased access to ancillary services.

Joining a group also has drawbacks:

- Some providers are less comfortable in a group setting and yet feel they have no choice but to join;

- Occasionally providers who have previously worked together will not all be invited to join a particular group, which often creates personal and professional anxiety for the individuals affected;

- Management decisions are no longer strictly in the purview of the physicians;

- Practice styles may not be compatible;

- Staff members who have worked with the group long term may not be retained in the new organization;

- All of the problems do not go away—new ones are constantly cropping up;

- Expectations are not met.

As groups form and professional management is in place, the fundamental differences in style and training between administrators and physicians shape the culture under which the formation will occur. Traditionally, the following factors have spawned unrest in these relationships:

- Physicians are trained to be independent. Most have enjoyed this aspect of practicing medicine and thus are reluctant to give it up. Managers, on the other hand, most often participate with teams and are more consensus builders than independent decision makers.

- Physicians have practiced in an environment where quick decision making is not only the norm, it is often critical to patient outcomes. Managers have traditionally done studies as issues arise and before taking any decisive action. These are key behavioral differences.

- Patients and others have long recognized physicians as authorities. Managers, on the other hand, have practiced in an information sharing mode and are generally not seen as authoritarian. They do, however, have high control needs, so the messages they send can get a bit mixed.

- Neither is particularly strong at fully appreciating the experience, knowledge and skills the other brings to the table. A great deal of time is spent trying to align behaviors. Time would be better spent appreciating the perspectives that they bring and working through the issues to reach common interest.

The physicians who are experiencing the most comprehensive changes are those who have had premanaged care practices. They are having to adapt to systems that were never a part of their overall approach to doing business during the bulk of their careers. They often do not have the systems in place to analyze the impact of managed care and/or to maximize their participation in this type of care delivery. Physicians in smaller groups who do not have a large base over which to spread the expenses of the information and tracking systems also are at a disadvantage in this rapidly changing environment.

PERCENT	AGE RANGES	COUNT
19%	Under 34	144,467
30%	35 - 44	225,858
21%	45 - 54	152,405
13%	55 - 64	96,049
17%	65 & Over	122,585

Source: Medsource, St. Paul, Minnesota 1995

Physicians over the age of 54 (30 percent in practice today) often started their practices and have had active, fully accountable roles in them for many years. They have practiced during a time when reimbursement was at its highest levels. At this career stage, they may wish to have more free time and are dealing with other life transformation issues, e.g., the kids are grown, life should be more fun, etc. Not trained to work in the market that faces them, they are apt to experience high levels of disillusionment. At a time when they should be looking forward to a higher income and less hassle, they are faced with just the opposite. They may move to organizational structures to attempt to provide some stability and support that they can no longer achieve practicing solo or in small groups. Their motivation, as they move to new structures, is not from a desire to change, but a defensive measure. The Sacramento-El Dorado Medical Society is seeking a consultant to study the degree of physician "burnout" and pursuing recommendations to put the joy back into practicing medicine. Transitions are difficult. Physicians in virtually every segment of the country will attest to increased stress within their practices.

Let us see, we are trying to build partnerships between parties who are not particularly enthusiastic about one another, have limited levels of trust, have very different perspectives on the world, bring different skills, have different management styles, and are often operating from a defensive as opposed to an offensive or neutral mind set. Is it any wonder greater than 80 percent of the ventures fail outright or dramatically fall below expectations?

Through understanding the behavioral and the structural issues, you will have a better chance than most to succeed. The key is to bring your colleagues and partners toward achieving the vision, educating them along the way, pointing out problems early and not losing your commitment to the process.

Independent Practice Associations

Because the lexicon is still evolving in the newly forming market, there are a variety of definitions for each term. The following definitions will be used for this discussion:

Independent Practice Association (IPA). An IPA is a corporation formed by physicians who maintain their independent practices but participate in the IPA to secure managed care business. IPAs accept financial risk for their members through capitation or discounted fees. The group is spread out geographically and is less formal than a group or staff model HMO. The only association between IPA providers is an individual contract between the physicians and the insurance company.

These models seek to preserve the autonomy of independent practice while providing a way for physicians to coalesce and deal with managed care providers. This is a delicate balance indeed. As competition heats up and the entity attempts to increase its market share and net revenues, difficult decisions necessarily have to be made. At times, the IPA (which often has a "dismissal without cause" clause) may exclude certain providers who are not performing up to the managed care standards necessary to meet payer demands. This causes concern among the regular members and leads to apprehension about "who is next to be excluded?" Further, as physicians participate more strongly in the management of any of these models, it is common for their colleagues to feel they have lost touch with the "practicing physicians" and to begin to distrust them.

IPAs may consist of multiple specialties or a group of single specialties. IPAs may consist of multiple specialties or a group of single specialties. Many analysts believe this model will prove to be superior to many others and are quickly surpassing the Group Practice Without Walls structure. Typically, they do not cost a lot to capitalize, though when the association discusses cost, the significant "sweat equity" of the physicians tends to be overlooked. The main need for capital comes if the IPA decides to invest in a shared information system. Shared information systems, and the people to work with them, cost from $250,000 to $1,000,000 or more. The investment must come from the physicians themselves unless they have secured capital support from a related hospital. If so, some significant issues arise for both parties regarding for-profit and not-for-profit status, private inurement and similar matters. If one partner is not a physician, carefully consider the tax consequences of this "new" IPA strategy on the front end of the deal. Keep in mind that the physicians must finance a physician-only structure. Once you begin to accept financial support from other entities, you have begun to change your base of control over decision making. Perhaps you are beginning to tread on less safe ground as seen not only by the Internal Revenue Service, but the Federal Trade Commission, who monitors antitrust. Both issues will be discussed in a later section.

Beginning a successful IPA requires facing several barriers. They are similar to the problems encountered in any number of ventures involving new partners and differing agendas.

- *A shared vision is essential,* not only for the "manager types," but for the organization to know where it is going and to defuse "us" versus "them" struggles that inevitably arise. This can be one of the most difficult steps and can quickly seem irrelevant to the "business of getting on with the business." Nevertheless, you will find taking the appropriate time with this step pays off when issues arise down the line and the startup is not going smoothly. Never take a trip without knowing where you are going.

- *Differences*—real or perceived—in "core values." As the parties begin to articulate their values, one party inevitably accuses another party of being more concerned with the money than the patients. If that is truly the case, you should perhaps reconsider this connection. More often, these perceptions are the result of poor communication and increasing levels of frustration among group members. It is not a bad idea to hire a facilitator who will keep the group on track yet does not have a business interest in the deal. This facilitator should not be a current member of any of the groups or of the hospitals. Many consultants are available to help you with this one.

- ***Lack of data*** to evaluate the most appropriate structure and the impact the group will have on the market. Gathering data is time consuming and can be expensive. The American Medical Association, Medical Group Management Association (MGMA), your professional societies and a variety of seminars can help you with this. In the final stages, though, you must compare your local data with communities of like size, consider the variables you deal with day-to-day and determine the structure most likely to take you toward your vision. Talking with local major employers regarding how they see the health care market for their employees over the next two to five years can yield some excellent data. This will also give you an opportunity to closely interact with a potential buyer of your services.

- ***Failure to agree in the early stages:***

  - how (specifically) the association is to be governed; how new members of the board will be selected; how non-board members interact with the board and management;

  - how the income will be distributed among the group and between primary care (and specialists, if applicable);

  - what the capital needs are anticipated to be in the first three years and how to fund them;

  - what the management structure will be; how the management will be selected; how much of their salary will be "at risk" based on incentives; how many layers of management does the organization need and is willing to support.

At least two publicly traded companies have IPA management as their primary line of business. They are FPA Medical Management and AHI Healthcare Systems. In addition, several investor-owned management companies also provide IPA management services.

When you are considering management candidates, be sure to follow these guidelines:

- Keep the name(s) of applicants confidential and only contact references after you have agreed on the timing. (You can hamper a person's career growth in this highly competitive time if current employers find their manager is looking at other opportunities.)

- Always check references and probe at least one or two layers deeper than the reference list suggests. To do this, when you are speaking to the listed reference, ask for the names of one or two others who can probably comment on this person's performance.

- Check with managed care companies with whom this person has negotiated in the past to determine what level of skill is present. Try to detect if there were problems between the managed care organizations and the candidate, including personality and style issues.

- Be on the safe side and get a release signed by the manager candidate permitting you to check any references. (This release is probably similar to ones you have signed to apply for hospital privileges or to participate in a managed care plan.)

- Determine why they left or are interested in leaving their last position.

- Consider running a check on criminal history to include convictions for Driving Under the Influence (DUI).

- If you will be advancing money for a signing bonus or relocation allowance, have the person sign a promissory note for the money. This will enable you to get all or part of your money back in the event the candidate does not come to work or does not stay in the job for a predetermined amount of time (unless you decide to terminate him).

- If you offer a letter of intent or contract before completing the reference checking, include a statement saying, "The agreement is good pending satisfactory reference checks."

- Be clear about the job description and your expectations of this manager, including the span of control.

If you are considering engaging a management company, be sure to follow these recommendations:

- Obtain a list of all IPAs the company has managed over the last three years.

- Look at their track record for retaining business.

- Talk with some management and nonmanagement physicians and nonphysicians who are being or have been managed by this company.

- Ask for the general terms they have negotiated for their IPA members and have them compare it with the terms others have garnered in the same market.

- Interview the person who will be the on-site manager (if there is one) or the management person with whom you will be interacting. Though you may not check references on them to the degree suggested above, you should make certain to design a thorough interview to determine compatibility with the style and values of the group.

- Obtain biographical sketches on the company's management personnel. Look at their experience within their current organization and whether they have had experience in other companies/markets.

- Clearly understand the management fees and try to negotiate to have the company "at risk" for compensation along the same lines physicians are at risk in the delivery of care. Even if you are unable to establish this arrangement, to go through the discussion and learn how the company views shared risk compensation arrangements will be good for you. Do they seem to have confidence in their ability to manage your group successfully? If so, a mutual risk arrangement seems worthwhile.

The formation and management of your IPA are big business. Do not spend less time in the early stages than you would if you were starting a new enterprise upon which your personal income rests. In the final analysis, what you are doing is exactly that.

Physician Organizations

"Hospitals have identified integration as a priority more out of an internal agenda that is centered around their survival. It's an agenda that strives to maintain the survival of hospitals under their current construct when, in fact, that construct is not going to exist. It is like coming up with a solution to yesterday's problem."

> — *Steve McDermott*
> *CEO, Hill Physicians Medical Group*
> *San Ramon, California*

Physician Organizations (POs). *Physician Organizations (POs) are models formed by and between groups of physicians. They take the same general shape and have the same goals as PHOs, but do not include the hospital as a partner. They vie for business with insurance companies and employers. They can subcontract work to one or more hospitals and can negotiate, en masse, for a preferred rate. They require a fair amount of capital and may have too narrow a service offering over time to be sustainable as an independent organization.*

(Physician Organizations can and do form partnerships with hospitals in a variety of ways. In order to be a Physician Organization as opposed to a Physician Hospital Organization, physician should form as a PO first and then contract with other entities.)

Physician organizations are excellent models for physicians to begin learning to work together while taking a relatively low risk look at the market's intricacies and the nuances of teaming with unfamiliar partners. Because they comprise solely physicians, no large partner is available to help with the capitalization needs, even to have the legal documents drawn and executed. They will also need capital for management and other types of support services if the group attempts to compete for managed care business strongly.

Physician Organizations are similar to IPAs, but they are usually not structured as tightly in the initial phases. The greatest challenge confronting a Physician Organization is to structure it as a unit to provide single signature contracting and/or to meet the needs of its members and the managed care contracting organizations through administrative efficiencies. Managed care organizations are seldom interested in groups that may splinter easily or cannot commit based on a single signature. Successful, mature Physician Organizations have met these challenges.

When they achieve this level of organization, the PO is indeed a Managed Care Organization with all the contracting opportunities and obligations of other models.

The Physician Organization must support and develop a strong physician leader who can devote sufficient time to the organization and management of the PO and handle a variety of contractual issues. Generally, the organization also needs the services of an attorney.

Because members of the hospital's traditional medical staff often form the PO, they frequently do not pay close enough attention to excluding members who are not suitable performers in a shrinking payment system. They are often overbalanced with specialists and take "any willing provider." This dilutes the volume of patients needed in each individual practice to encourage long term behavior changes.

Physician organizations often move into PHOs, IPAs or Integrated Delivery Systems (IDSs) over time. They do so, however, with more experience and understanding of the difficulties ahead than physicians who have not previously participated in any organizations competing for managed care business.

Group Practice Without Walls

Group Practice Without Walls (GPWW). In a Group Practice Without Walls, physicians align to contract with managed care companies as a group. The key to the success of this plan is strong alignment and centralizing administrative functions while maintaining independent office locations. Legal and financial requirements for forming a GPWW vary by region. They should be thoroughly investigated before deciding to form this type of entity. Additionally, reduction of administrative costs and centralization of administrative functions often means staff in individual offices must be moved or not retained. The political and financial consequences of these decisions should be thoroughly examined. If the groups are unwilling to reduce their administrative overhead, they will not maximize the benefit of this arrangement.

Group Practices Without Walls were originally formed to furnish solo practitioners and those in smaller groups with the benefits of being in a group practice while maintaining their individual offices and practice styles. This enables the physician to be part of a larger business in order to compete more effectively in the market. They were also originally formed to be wholly owned by physicians. Though there are wide geographical variances, in many parts of the country, the GPWW model has virtually faded from the integration scene and is rarely utilized today.

Physician Led MSOs and Physician Driven Provider Networks

"Integrating an organization actually is not hard. All you have to do is get a battalion of lawyers and health care consultants together and pay hundreds of thousands of dollars. Then, in three to six months, you'll have a contract that says you are integrated."

> — *David Ottensmeyer, M.D.*
> *Consultant (former CEO, Lovelace Industries*
> *Albuquerque, N.M.)*

The structures of MSOs and provider networks have previously been discussed. The leadership of the organization(s) does not dictate its structure, but may indeed dictate its success or failure.

Planning for and leading the organizations of the future will depend upon responding to the needs of the health care market. The planning tools of the past, which have largely been designed and driven by nonphysicians, will not be reliable guides to the future. Further, a critical requirement for success is the ability to vision a care system that is not based on past performance and "rules." It is innovative in how services are delivered and packaged to patients, payers and employers. This innovation cannot be undertaken by concentrating only on the payment mechanisms and the contractual relationships. The culture in which patient care is dispensed and disbursed will be largely driven by the physicians providing the care. They must have key decision-making roles.

It is physicians, not administrators, who will continue to be responsible for delivering the product to the market. It is physicians who will define value at the point of contact with the patient and understand the need to provide convenient services across a continuum of care.

However, a role exists for the trained nonphysician executive. Indeed, it will take a strong working relationship of many talented individuals and groups to make this all work. It is, however, key that physicians have significant roles in the design and delivery of products and that the clinical decisions do not become secondary to the financial decisions. They must balance to the needs of the market.

Physician-driven and provider-driven are different. Physician-driven is self-explanatory. Physicians largely make the decisions and they bring the product to market. Provider-driven refers not only to physicians, but to physician organizations, managed care organizations, hospitals, systems and the like. The provider of care, in this use, refers to clinic, hospital and outpatient settings and to the "trappings" that surround and support the care of the patient through a continuum. Physicians are not "just" providers, they are physicians. They are key components to a provider network. However, this network comprises more than the physician component. A provider network is a blend of the insurance side of the business and the clinical decision-making components of care.

The successful MSOs and provider driven organizations of the future (and there will not be many of them) will depend upon physicians and hospitals and other market segments working in totally new ways. No longer can they defend their turf and only attend to their own agendas. The acrimonious relationships, no matter how they are pushed underground, must end and they must embrace a new focus, beginning with looking at market needs and demands. The parties must work "backwards" to determine the roles of the players.

Today's system largely works on the issues of control. The physicians and hospitals cannot balance the needs for more patient access through managed care contracts, keeping beds filled and maintaining the reimbursement rates of the past five years. Those days are over. History does not change quickly, however. The innate need to defend what has worked in the past looms as a key stumbling block to moving toward the future.

If the physician component is left out, all you will have is contracts and conflict. Neither of these does anything to change the culture and provide the care systems that patients and payers are demanding. Similarly, unless physicians work with the hospitals for the times when the patient needs that level of care on the continuum, the hospitals will not be there to provide efficient, high quality inpatient care.

The model that adequately rewards cooperative work will enjoy more success than one that depends on a "win-lose" scenario. If one party is to be successful, all must be successful. Otherwise, we may have desegregation on the surface, but we will be light years away from integration.

Traditionally, the business leadership has come from administrative executives. Rare are the physicians who are prepared to fulfill these roles. Physicians are often able to lead other physicians, but perhaps have difficulty in determining where they ultimately want to end. The final destination is the result of hard work and a well-articulated vision that includes physicians and other providers.

A difference exists between management and leadership. Although these terms are often used interchangeably, they are really worlds apart. A manager is responsible for overseeing an operation and ensuring that certain tasks are performed according to a predetermined outcome. A leader is one who determines the outcome, decides what the final product should be, and persuades others to follow. Physician leadership is not well developed to work in today's health care environment and in the systems that will thrive over time.

A good deal of "bench strength" exists in the health care industry to accomplish the structural changes, reduce the legal exposure, provide tax planning, track costs, market programs, etc. The missing ingredient is physician leadership.

Far too many systems, hospitals and managed care organizations appoint physicians to high level roles without providing the support and tools required to lead the organization into the future. Though the organization may appear physician-driven and physician friendly on the surface, often it is not. Physician leaders may not be the hospital's "largest admitters," or they may not be the specialist who drives the most revenue into the managed care plan. They will be individuals with vision, who can influence change, communicate effectively and move an organization forward.

Physicians must play strong roles in determining the vision and culture of the organization(s) in which they participate. They are the culture to the patient, and best able to influence the vision and the process outcome. Not having physicians at the table playing active roles is folly when an organization is attempting to compete effectively in the market. Physicians will be interfacing directly with the patients. Thus, they will be able to influence the delivery of the product. Physicians serve as the "face of the organization" through more points of contact than any marketing executive or strategic planner can hope to accomplish. Each time a patient member of a health plan visits a network physician, the reputation of that plan is on the line. Moreover, each positive experience will generate "word of mouth" marketing; each negative experience will undermine any previous steps forward. The physicians are the product. You may confirm this by asking anyone how their health care needs are handled. Most likely, they will tell you about "their" clinic and "their" doctor—not their managed care organization.

Health care is a local business. Ingenuity to move forward in new ways will originate from clinics and physician led organizations, not large bureaucratic organizations. If the individual physicians are not involved at a grass root level, the ability to understand the local market and to meet its challenges will be encumbered. Physicians in their individual offices control the cost, quality and satisfaction levels of their patients. The combination of the experiences of many local physicians will drive the system—not a system assuming to understand the market absent of practicing physician views, creativity and involvement.

Demonstrating value in a health care system includes cost, quality, management of resources, and clinical outcome measurements. These can only be proved by involving physicians in the entire set of considerations on how to meet market goals in these areas. The physicians, by virtue of their work, will determine the quality, cost, resource management, outcomes, etc. Just as a company may be able to produce superior quality scalpels, management may be able to develop the tools, yet none of this makes a difference until the physician is involved.

Setting clear, measurable and "trackable" goals and objectives will be important, both to the long term success of the venture and in the near term. Goals will demonstrate progress to those involved and indicate if changes are necessary, etc. Setting goals that are not driven by the physicians providing care is ultimately a weak strategy.

The governance of an organization(s), especially organizations made up primarily of nonphysicians, must listen and learn from practicing doctors who are creating the culture by which their organization will be known. Physicians should have a strong voice in governance issues that will ultimately influence the product, its packaging, its pricing, outcomes measurements and the like. Governing boards should hear from more than management regularly and have a mechanism to seek out practicing physicians for educational purposes — one more side of being partners.

Physician clinical leadership will be required to move from a system of illness-based care to a system focused on prevention. A look at the compliance issues with patients, the long term versus short term gains/losses in this conversion process will be necessary from both a clinical and a managerial view. The investments made today may not pay off for ten years or more. How will that be financed, tracked and measured unless a system develops long term partnerships with physicians, payers and employers? Physicians, again, must drive the system.

Physicians are being called upon to become business partners and assist in maximizing environmental changes. They are designated to control the use of technology and other services, develop clinical protocols for treating illness, building the infrastructure (i.e., information systems) and leading clinicians and nonclinicians through the maze of meeting both patient and market expectations.

"The scarcest asset available in health care organizations today is physician leadership, and if the objective is to incorporate the medical staff's agenda into the agenda of an integrated organization, then one must arrive at the strategy of building a very strong cadre of physician leaders, physician managers and physician executives."

> — *David Ottensmeyer, M.D.*
> *Consultant*

The case for physician leadership is solid and convincing. The identification and/or development of physician leaders is not.

To provide the leadership in physician-led or the "driven" in physician-driven, physicians will need to have a person or persons who can and will —

- Invest the time and energy necessary to creating the vision and seeing it through the many changes it will naturally have to face.

- Be a person who has the respect of his peers and works from a consensus, not a fear-based approach.

- Represent the need for clinical integration along with the business planning necessary — not force one over the other, but accomplish the integration of the two.

- Emphasize partnerships between physicians and other care providers and provider organizations leading to shared arrangements for governance and economic risk.

- Challenge the current leadership/influence groups in ways that provide more opportunity for change.

- Understand and use clinical resource management data in their decision-making process.

- Help the system to reevaluate the use of nonphysician providers when appropriate and not tied into traditional, existing barriers.

- Represent the practicing physician perspective to a variety of audiences to include not only their colleagues, but the employers, payers and other components of the health care market.

- Learn from new partners about their concerns and bring that learning back to their colleagues in a meaningful way that promotes unity and reduces division.

- Take risks—nothing in the new market is a sure thing. The physician leader must have enough self-confidence and political capital to make mistakes, learn from them and move forward without losing his following.

- Strive to balance the interests of primary care and specialists by focusing on the needs of the market instead of the needs of the current system.

- Appreciate and not be disillusioned by ambiguity and conflict.

- Develop and use strong negotiating skills and learn to bargain from a base of shared interests among all involved parties.

- Listen.

- Challenge.

- Build a consensus.

- Demonstrate integrity of purpose during times of debate and disagreement.

- Have a keen interest in the welfare of the patient above all else and yet understand there are multiple ways to serve the patient of today and the patient of tomorrow.

Choosing physician leaders to follow is the last place for any hint of the "good old boy" network, the he/she-has-the-time-he/she-can-do-it system, the patronage system of the past, the selection of the angriest or loudest no matter how much they want to lead. Physicians will be looked to for leadership. The selection of the "spokespersons" or "spokes groups" will define that leadership in the eyes of multiple partners. Choose or volunteer wisely.

On the other hand, physicians who are leaders may not always have the skills necessary to operate most effectively in the nonclinical arena. They will often need development in the following areas:

- Understanding health systems structured under hospitals and managed care organizations, etc.

- Interpreting market and financial data sets.

- Management theories that are operating elsewhere in the market.

- Awareness of the market forces locally and elsewhere in the country.

- The range of integration models that are in use today and contemplated for the future.

- The history of how your market got to where it is today and interpretation of that data into meaningful bits of information to begin growing a new system.

- The expectations and agendas of their colleagues and new partners.

This last bullet point is especially important. Physician and nonphysician leaders most often fail because they do not know what is expected of them. For example, if a physician leader's constituencies expect protection from the unpleasant market changes and are unclear about that (unrealistic) expectation, there will be no opportunity for discussion of what is possible and impossible and what the leader can and cannot be expected to accomplish before they deem that person a miserable failure and another is selected (often likely to follow the same course). If the new partners expect the physician leader to "keep the doctors happy," he should know about that expectation. He should receive some education about the desirability and potential of that happening given the tasks at hand, before he is deemed to have "lost control of the troops" and regarded as a miserable failure.

Physician leaders should receive information and/or training in areas where they are less accomplished. To gain this information, they should be encouraged to develop mentoring relationships with those outside the clinical realm. Their colleagues and/or partners should support their development by providing the time, finances and tools for them to climb the learning curve. Simultaneously, nonphysician leaders must invest in learning how physicians think, what are their concerns, etc. The new partnering does not simply consist of the physician venturing into the world of new business and legal concepts, but also nonphysicians venturing into the world of care delivery. By this, they better understand the product they are attempting to develop together. Strategic and financial investment in leadership is never a waste. It not only yields stronger leaders, it also forces the parties to be more supportive and patient with those who are traveling on new ground.

Physicians are in the best position to understand the delivery system, change provider behavior and track clinical outcomes in "real time." Directly or indirectly, physicians control the system. They must couple that position with the leadership that will make it work best in the new era.

Case Examples

Following are some examples of physician led MSOs and provider networks:

- Albert Barnett, M.D., in 1988 tried to interest a hospital partner in providing inpatient care for his medical group's enrollees. He found these hospital executives were not ready to move from their traditional roles of filling beds and defending current revenue positions. While this may be understandable, it was unacceptable and as a result, the Friendly Hills Health Care Network purchased La Habra Community Hospital to form the Friendly Hills Regional Medical Center. They are now considering purchasing a second hospital to accommodate their growth. Barnett attributes their success to being able to capitalize on the economies and synergies needed to operate effectively in a managed care environment. Hospital executives, in his experience, "keep on trying to run the same old business." This is truly a health system run by physicians who not only direct the care but also create the culture.

  Friendly Hills, known as one of the most innovative networks in the country, was acquired by Caremark International. As of this writing, MedPartners/Mullikin is positioned to acquire Caremark creating the second-largest active physician group in Southern California reflecting the consolidation of medical groups throughout California and the nation overall. If this merger is completed, the new entity would be called MedPartners, Inc. These physicians have done an exemplary job of leveraging their positions and providing leadership in providing high quality managed care.

- American Health Network, centered in the Midwest, owns physician practices in Indiana, Ohio and Kentucky. Standing currently at 210 physicians, it expects to nearly double its size in 1996. It is run by physicians and based on the theory that continuity of care is key to controlling costs and promoting quality. It believes that if not for the fluid nature of today's population (e.g., job changes, geographic changes, employer benefit plan changes, etc.), people would largely remain with one physician indefinitely.

  American Health Network contracts with any managed care organization or insurer and multiple hospitals. It is a risk bearing organization, which makes it attractive to managed care organizations. Its lack of primary affiliation with any single hospital or hospital system makes it attractive to patients, and its multiple hospital affiliations not only meet the market demands but leaves the network able to negotiate for inpatient care. Physicians hold an ownership position in the company. There are currently plans to take the network "public" in the next two years.

- The Mayo Clinic is working with IBM and John Deere, both Fortune 500 companies, to develop managed care products cooperatively, thus increasing the potential of capturing large blocks of patient referrals.

- In September 1994, the Lahey/Hitchcock clinic resulted from the merger of two large multi specialty groups in New England. The merger produced the third-largest group practice in the country at that time, with 800 physicians.

As the pace of change accelerates, more mergers between unlikely partners are emerging, investing, divesting and metamorphosing into a wide range of organizational structures. The physicians are seeing many market initiatives by competitors such as home health care agencies, rehabilitation, long-term care facilities, and a variety of alternative therapies. To only consider competition from hospitals and managed care organizations is a short-sighted approach. The market is heating up, and the definition of who will be playing is constantly changing.

As a physician, look for the following basics in considering your entry into any organization whether they call themselves physician led, physician driven or any other of a number of "market driven" phrases:

- ***What does the organization mean by physician-led or physician-driven?*** In asking this question, you will be able to ascertain whether the organization's view of the role of physicians are compatible with your view.

- ***How are decisions made?*** Find out what kind of decisions physicians or full partners are making, ranging from the selection of management to organizational structural changes, to the type and number of contracts that they will enter.

- ***Meet the physician leaders.*** Can the organization show a commitment to physician leadership both in the selection of the leader(s) and their development, or is this simply an organization that has decided to "reward" an elder leader with the title and none of the "real" influence? Find out what this leader sees as the vision and what key strategies he thinks he will need to accomplish if the organization is to succeed.

- ***Who comprises the governing board and how are the members selected?*** Though there will be some regulatory requirements, physician involvement on the board should be significant, either directly or through active (not figurehead) committees, advisory groups, etc.

- ***How does the organization accomplish its strategic planning process?*** Besides finding out who is involved, get a copy or executive summary of the plan if they can make one available. (Note, most organizations consider this plan proprietary, so you may not have much success.) Ask how the organization has performed against the plan for the past year.

- ***What is the vision of the organization?*** The people you are talking to should be able to articulate this vision without having to look it up—preferably not verbatim, but in a way that is credible and shows a strong level of commitment. What do you think about the vision? Is it realistic? Ask for a set of examples regarding how they plan to get from where they are to where they think they are heading. Find out how they derived the vision and who was involved. Be sure the vision is a working vision—not just existing for purposes of a marketing logo.

Be very careful if the vision has not been determined unless this is an extremely new organization or idea you are being asked to participate in building. A lack of vision generally converts into a lack of success.

- ***Determine the growth plans.*** A part of the vision may or may not pertain specifically to the issues of growth. This is an important question as it helps you look at how the organization may look in the coming months or years and lets you consider your competitive alternatives.

- ***What has been the financial performance? What pressures are brought to bear regarding financial indicators?*** Obviously, the financial performance of any organization you are considering affiliating with is important. In these organizations, however, because they are so new, it is even more important to see how they are currently doing, what the trend line is, how they are performing based on expectations and what plans they have to enhance their financial performance further. Since the office-based physicians are the keys to any organization trying to meet market demands, the strategies for financial performance will directly affect you, as an individual or small group. Know what they are.

- ***Reference the organization through its current members.*** Find out from practicing physicians in the organization how they feel about their affiliation and what they considered important in their decision to join. Ask what they think of the leadership and any other parties who may be involved. Find out if, all things being equal, they would join again. Be forthright in your questions and listen closely to the response. These practicing physicians are wearing the shoes you are considering wearing.

A thorough examination of a physician driven or physician led organization is no less important than an examination of a different model. Be sure the physician leadership is competent, active (not in title only) and being developed.

If you are interested in providing physician leadership and are applying for an administrative role, consider the following:

- ***Why do you want to do this?*** Many physicians, frustrated with the changes, are looking at the potential of a shift in their careers from hands on patient care to an administrator. If you are considering this approach as a defensive measure to protect your income and not as a true desire dramatically to change your role, your chances of success will be low and your frustration level may reach new heights.

- ***What skills do you have as a leader?*** Are you able to build a consensus and is that important to you? Can you work in team-based roles with physicians and nonphysicians? Do you value the participation of nonproviders of care in shaping the overall systems of the future? Do you have followers?

- *What new skill development will you require?* Not having the business and legal acumen required does not prohibit leadership, provided you can identify your weaknesses and commit to acquiring the knowledge necessary to shore up these weak spots. This may be done through formal training, through mentoring with others or through experience—it will generally be a combination of all three approaches.

- *Can you admit mistakes, make course corrections and move forward without dwelling on the "search for the guilty?"* An inordinate amount of time may be spent on trying to figure out who is at fault rather than acknowledging a problem and working cooperatively on its resolution. This is a luxury that the rapidly changing market will not extend.

- *What leadership do you want to provide?* Leaders are not always, in fact not often, paid executives. They are the physicians who are working with colleagues, serving patients and participating in building models. There are strong physician leaders in paid executive positions, but you do not have to hold one of these to provide leadership in a variety of segments of the emerging systems of care delivery. As you consider the potential opportunities available to you, decide how much time and energy you can commit to leading groups of people. The market is currently flooded with those who are seeking paid administrative and leadership posts and the industry is grossly neglecting the physician who is providing leadership day-to-day in the local clinics and communities. Obviously, title and leadership are not necessarily linked.

- *Are you prepared to go from the level of competence you now enjoy to a new field where you will not necessarily be recognized for your clinical skills?* This transition is often difficult for clinically based physicians. In their office settings, dealing with complex patient issues, they are self-assured and know what is to be done, how to do it and the steps to take next. Physician leadership, especially in this changing market, is not as straightforward. It requires risk taking, team building, relying on others and developing new skills. Many new physician leaders and managers find themselves personally uncomfortable with the "new kid on the block" role they are expected to assume, especially in paid positions. Those currently serving in recognized formal and informal leadership roles do not have the same pressures, as they are generally not radically changing their professional undertakings. Those moving to paid administrative positions often do not have the expectations clearly outlined and are working in a new arena where the "rules of the game," and indeed the game itself is often changing.

In considering leadership roles or any other of life's challenges, six steps can universally be counted on to emerge. They will not necessarily be in order, and you will visit many more than once in the life of the project. They are worth knowing.

Six Steps of Project Management

- Wild enthusiasm

- Mass confusion

- Disillusionment

- The search for the guilty

- The prosecution of the innocent

- The promotion of the uninvolved

Unfortunately, this list has stood the test of time. If you consider it closely against the challenges of wallpapering a room or trying to devise a new system of delivering health care services, you will find we vascilate between various points on the list. The frustrations are predictable and timeless. A bit of patience with emerging leaders and the process will be a fundamental requirement for success.

It has been said that leaders are born, not made. While this is not necessarily so, many characteristics lend themselves to leadership roles. Integrity and clarity of purpose, perhaps, lead the list, but being able to build consensuses, having skills in group dynamics, being able to lead and also follow, to talk and listen, to make mid-course corrections, to value the ideas of a variety of audiences, having patience, seeking understanding, avoiding self-interest, macro rather than micro managing and a strong sense of humor are not far behind.

CHAPTER 4

Nonproviders as Physician Organizers

Introduction

The person who is truly effective has the humility and reverance to recognize his own perceptual limitations and to appreciate the rich resources available through interaction with the hearts and minds of other human beings. That person values the differences because those differences add to his knowledge, to his understanding of reality. When we're left to our own experiences, we constantly suffer from a shortage of data....

The relationship of the parts is also the power in creating a synergistic culture inside a family or an organization. The more genuine the involvement, the more sincere and sustained the participation in analyzing and solving problems, the greater the release of everyone's creativity, and of their commitment to what they create.

— David Ottensmeyer, M.D.
Consultant

Because of the key physicians hold in making the health care system work (whatever its final structure), many groups are interested in organizing, partnering with, managing, controlling, merging with or otherwise affiliating with physicians. Physicians are bombarded with offers of "help" from various spectrums. Advice can come from physicians, hospitals, managed care organizations and practice management companies. Beginning with, "I'm from the government and I'm here to help you," through the adage of "Heaven helps those who help themselves," physicians (especially those in primary care) have never before been as ardently courted as potential partners as they are today.

Many views and skills are to be appraised. To find out what will be most effective for you and your market, compare your own vision of the future with those whom you will eventually partner and determine your potential for synergism.

In this section, we will look at two models of nonphysicians as physician organizers, managed care organizations and practice management companies. Both bring some value to the table. Both have tradeoffs. The discussion that follows should be beneficial in helping you decide which, if either, may be appropriate for you.

Managed Care Organizations

Managed care organizations are complex and structured in a variety of ways. (For extensive information on managed care, see *Managing Managed Care in the Medical Practice*, part of the *PRACTICE SUCCESS!©* *Series,* published by Coker Publishing and distributed by the American Medical Association, 1996.) The business of MCOs is to ensure the provision of high quality, cost efficient, accessible care to their members or enrollees. They accomplish this through a relationship or multiple relationships with physicians and other providers.

Managed care organizations may enter arrangements with physicians that include contracting for certain services through practice acquisition. Conventional managed care organizations are HMO's (Health Maintenance Organizations), IPAs (Independent Practice Associations) and PPOs (Preferred Provider Organizations).

Managed care organizations can bring substantial value to the table. For starters, they are generally well capitalized and can offer support services and organizational models, which are expensive to build on your own. They are "fluent in managed care and capitation" and therefore can lend their expertise and experiences in competing in today's market. They have data and experience in providing care efficiently, and they are clear in their focus on primary care. They offer a full gambit of services to members. The good ones have strong marketing and negotiating skills, bringing physicians increased access to groups of patients.

Some shortcomings become evident when managed care organizations begin to organize physician practices. Lack of expertise in running a medical practice is their primary weakness. Though business strengths generally abound in MCOs, they do not directly translate into the essential skills for building and maintaining a local practice. The MCO is often a large organization that may or may not be structured to offer support at an individual clinic or provider level. Business people working in the health care delivery system run MCOs, not physicians delivering care in the system. The difference in mentality between the business and the physician may pose too large a gap to span successfully. Further, the MCO's primary emphasis is on its relationship with the payer or employer, not the relationship between the physician and the patient. They focus on caring for populations instead of individual patients. That does not make their emphasis right and the physician's wrong, nor is the reverse wholly true. How well the MCO functions as a provider organizer and how well suited it is for the physician or practice will be determined by how well they blend their interests.

Sometimes, managed care organizations are acquiring practices to solidify their networks. Usually, they are buying primary care networks and contracting with specialists for the care of

their enrollees. They generally pay the specialists on a discounted fee-for-service basis while
they may pay the primary care physicians in a variety of ways, e.g., salary, salary plus
production, overall performance of the plan, etc. Most managed care organizations—except
closed panel models— allow their primary care networks to see patients from other MCOs to
provide the necessary volume to offset some overhead expenses. This is especially true while
MCOs are in the growth phase. They may not have a sufficient base of enrollees to support
the practices they have acquired.

Managed care organizations may serve as a continuum through which physicians can affiliate.
Though the terms may change, the basics are:

- *Associate.* At this level, there is limited if any integration between the parties. The
  relationship is based on some integration, primarily as a provider in the network who
  does not see many of the plan's patients.

- *Affiliate.* Physicians at this level may see a significant number of patients in the
  plan but also see other plan's patients; they do not integrate with the MCO to any
  large degree.

- *Partner.* Integration relationships are larger than any of the two above. The physicians
  may see more than 50 percent of their patients enrolled with the sponsoring MCO,
  participate in developing clinical guidelines and participate in activities that focus on
  achieving administrative efficiencies. This category would generally include members of
  the medical staff in any hospital(s) owned by the MCO.

- *Employed.* The MCO owns these physicians' practices and they employ the physicians.
  Though the physicians may see enrollees from other plans, they would have significant
  financial and administrative alignment.

Because of the competition for primary care and the need for specialists to span more than one
MCO or system, physicians can choose to affiliate in several ways. How much affiliation will
generally determine how much support the practice can expect from the MCO for staff and
provider training, access to services and electronic linkages. Relationships evolve over time. A
practice can enter at any point on the continuum and change their relationship based on
market conditions. As one begins to examine these affiliations, each party should clearly
understand the expectations of the other. Access to services of the MCO and the issues
surrounding terminating or changing the relationship over time should also be clear.

In considering being organized under an MCO, be sure to look at:

- ***The role of physicians within the MCO*** including any medical directors and/or associate
  medical directors. Do they have any role in the governance of the MCO? To whom do
  they report? What authority do they have? How do they interact with physicians in the
  network? How are disputes solved?

- ***How are clinical guidelines developed?*** Under whose direction is this task undertaken? How are the guidelines applied? Are they guidelines or are they mandates? What happens when they conflict with guidelines from another plan? Is there any effort made between physicians of various plans to standardize procedures?

- ***What "economic credentialing" data*** is gathered and what is done with it? Will you have access to the data on yourself? Who else will have that access and for what purpose? How are physicians handled who are outliers? Has the MCO ever separated from a physician over the economic data? If so, what was the consequence to each party?

- ***What is the satisfaction level of other physicians*** who are organized under this MCO? What is the reputation of the MCO in the community with payers and colleagues? What are the managed care contract retention rates? What has been the track record for acquiring new business? How are the contracts structured? Do the physicians generally get any withhold returned? Who are the salespeople in the field, and how are they marketing the network?

- ***What services you can expect and at what cost?*** Be sure the expectations are clear to both parties before you sign up.

- ***Can you participate in seeing patients of other managed care plans?*** This is especially important for specialists and large multi specialty groups. What are the issues for the MCO you are considering, and do the competitive MCOs have any "rules" against contracting with you if you are organized under this structure?

In many markets, organizing under a managed care plan is a good move. Gauging this decision against your own environment is important, however, and determines what is best for you.

Practice Management Companies

"This is a trillion-dollar cottage industry, and there isn't that much good management in health care. I think it's a great opportunity for investors. In many respects, we're looking at the HMO industry reborn; these [companies] are what HMOs were back in 1983."

— *Tom Hodapp*
Robertson, Stevens & Co.
San Francisco, California
Reported in Money and Management, Frank Cerne,
Vol. 69, Hospitals and Health Networks, 1/5/95.

A new development in the practice management scene is Investor Owned (Medical Practice) Management Companies (IOMCs), also called equity models and for-profit management companies. These companies generally purchase the nonprofessional assets of the practices (e.g., accounts receivable, equipment, leasehold improvements, etc.) and enter a long term management contract for the medical practice. This gives the IOMC the exclusive right to manage the practice for between 20-40 years, depending upon the terms negotiated. The nonprofessional employees become employees of the IOMC.

The IOMC generates revenue through practice management fees. The IOMC may purchase the nonprofessional assets of the clinic with cash, shares of restricted common stock and/or adjustable convertible debentures. (Convertible debentures are interest-bearing debt instruments that can be converted into stock in lieu of cash when they mature, typically over about four years.) Most IOMCs, but not all, have physicians as "owners." They also have some venture capitalists who help bring in the initial assets to get started who are also owners.

The IOMC is a stand alone business. It attempts to take a fragmented system of providers and weave it together without incorporating other partners, such as hospitals or insurers. These equity models generally mimic the independent practice of physicians in stronger ways than affiliation with other market forces. The physicians, especially as owners, participate heavily in the management and strategic planning of the individual clinic at the local level. They also have a strong interest in the overall success of the IOMC as stockholders. These models can satisfy the quest for autonomy and the need for a corporate partner.

The IOMC manages the cash flow, and when the company benefits, the physicians benefit through their stock. As IOMCs expand their networks nationally they can take advantage of a much larger market and a variety of managed care contracting vehicles. They have more diversified payor sources than those who are operating in smaller markets. They can depend upon a large network of providers in dissimilar geographic and business markets to strengthen and stabilize the company. These companies operate in multiple states and take advantage of indemnity payers and managed care contracting opportunities. Nashville-based PhyCor, for example, is currently operating in or has acquisitions pending in 20 states. No single clinic or market contributes more than 15 percent of its revenues. They are generally very strategic in their growth plans and enter markets selectively, often beginning where managed care plays a small part in the market. They use multiple strategies for internal growth to increase volume at the local clinics and thus increase productivity.

Though investor-owned companies currently account for only 2 percent of the total group practice revenues, predicted growth over the next five years is 13.5 percent. The market capacity is an estimated $64 billion.

Two prototypes dominate the equity models. One model manages large multi specialty group practices; the other has a more narrow approach on a single specialty. PhyCor, MedPartners/ Mullikin and Caremark currently dominate the market in multi specialty practices. Firms primarily involved in single specialty arenas are American Oncology Resources, Physician Reliance Network and OccuSystems, among others. Single specialty companies rely on their ability to provide appropriate levels of specialty care to managed care enrollees, with more cost-efficiency than independent or PHO specialist groups. This requires a high level of discipline and alignment of financial incentives, both of which are present in equity model companies.

Clarity of focus is probably the major difference between these models and other previously discussed models. Equity model companies concentrate their efforts in managing physician practices in diverse markets. They are not concerned with filling hospital beds; in fact, they can often leverage better pricing from hospitals since they have no particular business ties in communities that have multiple competing inpatient hospital units. They are not concerned with referrals to specialists. Neither are they necessarily concerned with supporting high levels of technology, nor with affiliating with the local medical school. They manage physician practices, keep the physician in an independent, yet involved, role and build a strategically diverse market.

These organizations have enamored the Wall Street financial market, and their yields have been particularly strong. The three largest, PhyCor, Coastal and Pacific Physician Services, are enjoying annual earnings growth of more than 30 percent. Any investment dealing with a sector of health care is unpredictable given the market turmoil. These companies, however, seem to be providing a marketable product as they bring their physicians' expertise into a variety of markets.

Questions continue concerning the long term ability of these equity models to be the ultimate organizers of physician practices. Clearly, they are growing fast and acquiring many practices. What the future (e.g., the 15th and 20th years) of the contractual arrangements will hold is anyone's guess. Skeptics predict the increasing pressure to maintain the strength of the stockholder's earnings per share will cause physicians to lose their enthusiasm for these models. This has not happened yet.

If you are considering entering these models, the tables on the next few pages should give you some valuable information.

Beyond reviewing the prospectus and the gleaning information from marketing brochures, consider doing the following research:

- Do a literature search on three or four of the companies in which you are interested. Write and ask them for an annual report and a listing of their clinics. Call some physicians and find out what their experience has been.

- Follow the stock market over time to help understand the earnings trends. Find out why the shares are earning what they are; follow new acquisitions and look at their market diversification.

- Do not lose sight of your local needs. Collaboration with other local resources will ultimately be key to the services that providers can deliver in your community. Never underestimate the current competition or that which they may bring in if you join a management firm that will not work with the hospitals and employers in your area. They will not idly stand by and relinquish their interests. What may seem like a captive market today could be radically different with the recruitment of new physicians to the community, the closure of your local hospital, the exodus of specialists or the "lock out" by major employers.

- Keep an eye on legislative trends in your state. Your local and national medical societies and the AMA play key roles in the provision of health care. They also have a good deal of lobbying strength. The rules under which you operate today can and probably will change.

- Always remember you are part of your community. The perception of those constituents continues to be very important in your future as a physician and as a member of the local milieu. Though the provision of health care has a strong business element, enterprise is not the sole consideration in determining the best structure for you and your practice.

Public Companies

Company	Ticker	Physicians	Model Type
American Oncology Resources	AORI	148	Single Specialty (Oncology)
Caremark#	CK	1,100	Multispecialty
Coastal Physician Group#	DR	220	Primary Care
Equivision**	EQVN	103	Specialty (67 Opthamology and 36 Oncology)
FPA Medical Management#	FPAM	100	Primary Care
Health Care & Retirement#	HCR	25	Single Specialty (Opthamology)
InPhyNet#	IMMI	120	Primary Care
MedCath#	MCTH	64	Multispecialty & Cardiology
MedPartners/Mullikin@	MPTR	1,200	Multispecialty
OccuSystems	OSYS	128	Single Specialty (Occupation Health)
Pacific Physicians Services*	PPSI	310	Primary Care (focus on primary care)
Pediatrix#	PEDX	116	Single Specialty (Pediatrics)
PhyCor	PHYC	1,900	Multispecialty
Physicians Resource Group	PRG	256	Single Specialty (Opthamology)
Physicians Reliance Network	PHYN	203	Single Specialty (Oncology)
Theratx#	THTX	100	Single Specialty (Occupational Health)

Private Companies

Company	Physicians	Model Type
Allied Physicians, Inc.	128	Multispecialty
American Opthalmic	70	Single Specialty (Opthamology)
First Physician	60	Multispecialty (focus on primary care)
GynCor, Inc.	14	Single Specialty (Infertility)
Health Partners	100	Multispecialty (focus on primary care)
PRIMECARE	261	Primary Care

**Assumes completion of pending merger with 30 oncology centers with 36 oncologists

*Under agreement to be acquired by MedPartners/Mullikin

@Assumes completion of acquisition Pacific Physicians

Physician equity model physician practice management not sole source of company income

Source: Company Data

Physician Practice Management Industry – January 11, 1996

Company Name	FY	Symb	1/10/96 Price	52-Wk. Hi	52-Wk. Lo	Yld.	FY EPS 1994	FY EPS 1995	FY EPS 1996	CY EPS 1995	CY EPS 1996	CY P/E 1995	CY P/E 1996	Mkt. Val. (Mil)	3-Yr. Proj. LTG	Rating	Analyst
Business &Processing Services																	
Medaphis Corporation	12	MEDA	35.75	41	20	0.0%	0.54	0.81	1.06	0.81	1.06	44.1	33.7	1,645	35%	1	Carpenter,C.
Information Systems																	
IDX Systems Corp.	12	IDXC	29.75	35	23	0.0%	0.18	0.54	0.62	0.54	0.62	55.1	48.0	586	30%	2	Gallo, A.
Medic Computer Syst., Inc.	12	MCSY	62.25	70	31	0.0%	0.94	1.32	1.72	1.32	1.72	47.2	36.2	710	30%	1	Gallo, A.
Nursing & Long-Term Care																	
Health Care & Retirement Corp	12	HCR	34.13	36	25	0.0%	1.26	1.55	1.85	1.55	1.85	22.0	18.4	1,130	20%	1	Swenson, J.
TheraTx, Inc.	12	THTX	10.13	23	10	0.0%	0.75	0.98	1.20	0.98	1.20	10.3	8.4	211	25%	3	Swenson, J.
Other Services																	
Physician Sales & Service, Inc.	3	PSSI	22.50	29	6	0.0%	0.09	0.11	0.32	0.25	0.41	90.0	54.9	783	40%	1	Ryan, B.
Pharmaceuticals-Special Situation																	
Henry Schein, Inc.	12	HSIC	24.25	30	20	0.0%	0.58	0.67	0.86	0.67	0.86	36.2	28.2	306	20%	2	Ryan, B.
Providers																	
American Oncology Resources	12	AORI	44.38	50	25	0.0%	0.08	0.49	0.95	0.49	0.95	90.6	46.7	1,012	35%	2	Kerns, E.
MedPartners, Inc.	12	MPTR	29.00	35	15	0.0%	(0.12)	0.37	0.77	0.37	0.77	78.4	37.7	502	35%	2	Kerns, E.
OccuSystems, Inc.	12	OSYS	17.75	22	16	0.0%	0.14	0.42	0.61	0.42	0.61	42.3	29.1	356	35%	2	Kerns, E.
PhyCor, Inc.	12	PHYC	39.25	51	18	0.0%	0.42	0.60	0.84	0.60	0.84	65.4	46.7	1,522	35%	1	Kerns, E.

ANALYSTS' STOCK RATING

Analyst Stock Ratings refer to our analysts' assessment of a stock's likely
Performance relative to the market over a six to twelve month time horizon:

(1) Strongest overperformance / Strong Buy
(2) Overperformance / Buy
(3) Market performance / Neutral

(4) Underperformance / Source of Funds
(5) Substantial underperformance / Sell
SR – Suspended Rating

CHAPTER 5

Necessary Tools for All Physicians

Understanding the Business of Physician Practice Management

The days are gone for counting on having a successful business simply through seeing patients and sending out invoices. Governmental regulations, reimbursement shifts and market pressures have moved medicine away from being a business with a primary focus on caring for one patient at a time. Now, practicing is an administrative nightmare comprising accounts receivable and collections management, and human resources management. It requires determining sources of capital, negotiating managed care contracts, and competing for the employee populations of major employers. Further, a practice has infinite needs for strong information systems, measuring outcomes and proving quality.

Practice management has become a big business. Most physician practices are having management difficulty, either because they lack the time or they lack the training, or, most likely, a bit of both.

Today's office setting must concern itself with regulatory compliance in the laboratory and radiology areas, compliance in coding and billing, quality assurance programs, risk management, accounts receivables, collections, negotiating contracts with third party payers and evaluating the risks associated with those contracts, patient satisfaction, data collection, financial tracking/trending and outcomes measurement. These represent many full time jobs and require considerable training and continuing education. Massive information system needs must be met. The selection of computer hardware and software and system maintenance and upgrading requires specialized training and recurring capital expenditures.

Besides business operations, human resources management demands compliance with wage and hour regulations, accommodation for the disabled in adherence with the Americans with Disabilities Act (ADA), staff selection and scheduling, hiring, training, discipline and termination of staff, as appropriate. Professional staffs (i.e., registered and licensed practical nurses) have state mandated scope of practice issues to meet.

Few physicians can successfully balance the complexities of the office business practice yet see enough patients to grow or maintain stability. Beyond the risks faced in managing patient care, significant financial risks are involved in managing the operational areas of the business.

Physicians need significant professional assistance to maximize the assets of their practice and to advise about decisions that may be costly. Many companies and consultants are available to help. In earlier sections, we discussed consultant selection and suggested ways to screen for basic concerns.

Before investing in a consultant, consider additional resources that may prove helpful and are reasonably priced or free. You may obtain names of quality ones through the American Medical Association, your state and local associations/societies, Healthcare Financial Management Association (HFMA) and the Medical Group Management Association (MGMA).

Physicians play the essential role in practice management, not only through seeing patients and providing the necessary clinical expertise, but mostly through establishing and exemplifying the culture of the clinic to employees, patients, partners and colleagues.

Physicians often do not realize their "clout" with staff members, with patients and their families, and in reaching other parts of the community. The physician who models a professional and positive attitude and accepts nothing less from his staff is managing the practice as no one else can.

Following are some tips to consider in managing the culture of the practice:

- ***Routinely conduct patient satisfaction surveys.*** Collect data from a wide range of patients who are exhibiting an extensive scope of clinical problems to capture a broad look at your patient population. Make sure your staff sees patient satisfaction surveys as important and that they politely follow up to ensure the information is collected.

- ***Have a system for following up on problems identified on your surveys and for tracking trends.*** Make certain your staff feels accountable for the outcome of the surveys along with the physicians.

- ***What do your patients see when they are in your office?*** Instead of entering your office through your private entrance, occasionally enter through the same door your patients use. Look at your waiting room and the conduct of your staff. Is the room clean and inviting? Are the staff members attentive to the patients and the business or discussing personal issues? You may learn some very important things about how it feels to be a patient sitting in your waiting room.

- ***Clear up attitudinal issues among members of your staff.*** Terminate personnel, if necessary, and hire people with a strong commitment to customer service. Think about where you do business, for example, as a consumer. Unless you are treated well, you will likely seek alternatives, even if the product is of high quality. Patients assume quality; they understand and demand courtesy.

- *Are your physician colleagues representing your practice in a way that reflects your attitudes?* If not, speak to them openly and forthrightly. Attempt to work together to make these important changes. If you are having difficulty with them, chances are others are too.

Do not view cultural issues as inconsequential. The relationships you build, individually and as a group, will carry your practice. They will make a difference as you strive to provide leadership and benefit you over time through the multiple business and professional partnerships you must build to meet today's market challenges.

Cost and quality will be "mandated" in one form or another. Differentiation will come as the delivery of service.

Know the Operational Strengths and Weaknesses of Your Practice

To assess the strengths and weaknesses of your particular practice, take a planned, candid look at the components of the operation. The following checklist should be useful. Add other issues that are pertinent to your particular market.

Physicians

- How many physicians are in your practice?

- Have you had difficulty retaining physicians in your practice? If so, find out why. Perhaps you are doing a poor job of initially selecting candidates, or maybe you have an internal problem causing them to relocate—either way, it needs to be fixed.

- Is this number sufficient to handle the current and anticipated patient load while allowing physicians to have some time away, take vacation, and cover a call schedule with reasonable comfort?

- How long are you/your partners planning to practice?

- What are your plans for recruiting physicians into the practice either as additional members or to replace a partner who may be reducing hours or retiring?

- What is your group's reputation within the general community? In the hospital? With managed care payers?

- Do you or your partners need additional training or to "brush up" on particular techniques that would enhance the overall service capabilities of the group? If so, how is this going to be handled?

- Do you or any of your colleagues have particular leadership skills that would enable them to assume a "lead" role? If so, how is their practice time to be replaced and how will the compensation (if any) for this leadership be handled (e.g., paid directly to the physician, paid to the practice to pay the replacement, etc.)

- Should any other specialities/specialists be brought into the practice or be subcontracted to serve your patient base and control costs? If so, what are the plans?

Support Staff

- How much professional support staff per physician do you have in your practice?

- How do your ratios compare with other clinics your size with your speciality or mix? (MGMA can give you statistical data for measurement.)

- What are the ratios of other clinics similar to yours in your community?

- Do you have staff turnover problems? If so, why?

- Who is the office manager for your group and what criterion was used to select this person for the job? Do they need additional education or development to do the job well? If so, what is the plan?

- Is there a difference between the "formal" leadership and the informal leadership? If so, is it a problem?

- Do you perform annual performance appraisals on your staff or arrange for someone to handle this? Are these reviews documented, signed and filed?

- Are your salaries for staff competitive within the market of like clinics? If you think so, how do you know?

- Do you "credit" people for years of experience and pay them accordingly? Are there internal equity issues?

- Are the benefits competitive with other clinics?

- Do you have a large accrual on the books for vacation or sick leave earned but not paid?

- What is the morale of your staff? How do you know?

- Does your staffing flex with the schedules of the physicians?

- What does the staff do when you and your colleagues are not in the clinic? What new things might they do?

- What are the systems they have established and/or follow for dealing with patient complaints, new business challenges, etc.? Do they feel a part of the clinic? Is this important work to them or just a job? Does it show?

- Do you have the right number of people? The right mix? How do your salaries compare as a percentage of overhead?

Contractual Arrangements

- What percentage of your business is through managed care contracts? What are the terms of these contracts? How likely is renewal?

- What is the practice's financial performance under these contracts?

- What data are you receiving individually and/or as a group regarding your performance? How does this compare with others in the plan(s)?

- What are the major employers in your community doing about controlling the cost of providing health care to their employees? Are they considering forming any type of coalition? If so, how do they plan to partner with you and/or your group? If you do not know, how can you find out?

Hospital Relationships

- What is the financial status of your local hospital?

- If more than one hospital is in your market, what are their cooperative and competitive plans? How can/should you and/or your colleagues be involved?

- What is the ratio of primary care physicians to specialists in your market? Whom do you refer to and why? What are their outcomes and cost efficiencies? Are the primary care groups and/or specialists forming coalitions? Will they invite you to join. Why or why not?

- How committed is the local hospital's management to redefining the provision of health care as opposed to filling beds?

- What is the cost of the local hospital compared with its nearest competitor? To national standards? Does this now or will it in the future affect your reimbursement?

- How is the quality of care being provided to your patients?

- Do the emergency room physicians treat patients with a managed care mindset?

- How amenable is the hospital and its medical staff to change?

Market/Competitor Analysis

- Is your population growing or shrinking?

- Who are the major employers and how stable are they?

- What are the age/gender demographics of the market?

- What managed care plans are operating in your market and are they growing?

- What are the particular arrangements of the plans?

- Is your clinic geographically located to provide patient access for employees and enrollees?

- Do you have or need to add an urgent care service?

- Is your clinic open at convenient times, i.e., evenings and weekends?

- What are the other clinics in town doing about hours, services and outreach programs?

- Do you have access to market data that will help you plan for the future?

Strengths, Weaknesses, Opportunities and Threats

Using the information you have gathered, a "SWOT" analysis of your clinic should help you determine how well you are positioned and what changes you may need to effect to remain competitive. Beyond the above data consider:

Strengths

- What is your clinic known for?

- How well respected are you in the community/with your colleagues?

- How broad is your referral base locally and in outreach areas?

- Can you differentiate based on service?

- Are your patient satisfaction surveys on a positive trend line?

Weaknesses

- Is your facility modern and up-to-date or will you need to seek access to major capital for improvements?

- Are your information systems strong enough to support your clinic? To interface with managed care plans? To gather the appropriate data to help you with strategic and business planning?

- Are you able to recruit for succession planning and/or to add new providers/services?

- Can you/should you utilize Physician Assistants and/or Nurse Practitioners to support your patient base?

- Have you been excluded from any managed care plans due to professional or economic credentialing issues?

Opportunities

- Are there niche markets not currently being met that you might enter?

- Should you consider forming or being part of a physician coalition, PHO, MCO, GPWW, IPA or other organizational structure? Why or why not?

- Can you provide leadership to meet market demands?

- Are there ways you can meet and work with major employers in the area on prevention issues, or "bulk" provision of patient care?

- Are you leading or following the market?

Threats

- Is your patient base diversified enough to withstand the loss of a particular enrollee or patient population?

- Are there competitors preparing to enter your market either through MCOs, new provider clinics, for-profit management companies and the like?

- Is your fee schedule competitive? When was it last updated?

- Are you in full compliance with state and federal regulations in your business practices?

- Are you being excluded from discussion or membership in any major plan or organization? If so, why? Is it something you can correct?

- Are you being paralyzed by anger or frustration?

By conducting a thorough analysis of your practice—the business you know best—and gleaning as much information as possible from your colleagues and competitors, you will be better able to execute course corrections to stay even or grow in the market. These analyses are not easy. They require you to step back and look at both your staff and infrastructure, and also your colleagues and yourself. You cannot carry extra baggage into the future. To maximize the opportunities before you and be able to move quickly requires having an efficiently running business. If you cannot make changes because you are tied to the past, either through your practices, staff or attitudes, you are at a distinct disadvantage in this turbulent market.

Obviously, merely gathering the data and taking the tough look is insufficient. Changes are necessary in almost any practice. The market has and is undergoing major changes—to believe you can stay the same and meet the needs of a changing market is unrealistic. Just as you consider Subjective and Objective data about your patients, and from that data determine your Approach and Plan, so will you need to look at your practice and your position in the marketplace.

This analysis should be considered and updated as appropriate. It should not be merely an exercise that captures your imagination for the moment and is not referenced until some magic annual cycle comes around. It should be a living document, complete with a vision statement that helps you find your direction and chart your course.

Knowing the Current Worth of Your Practice

As you consider the alternatives available to you, knowing the value of your current practice is important. The valuation of a practice in today's environment is under intense scrutiny by the Internal Revenue Services for potential private inurement and the Office of the Inspector General (IOG) for violations of federal anti-kickback statutes.

Several approaches may be taken to value a practice. Begin by obtaining an independent valuation for the practice by a Certified Public Accountant or consulting firm familiar with physician practice appraisals. Use the valuations as a basis for beginning your negotiations.

In this section, we will not attempt to describe the accounting methods for valuing a particular practice. An excellent article "Looking beneath the surface valuing health care intangible assets" by James G. Rabe, CFA, ASA, co-director of the Portland, Oregon, practice office of Management Associates is used as a resource for the information provided below. Further, comprehensive information is available through another volume in the *PRACTICE SUCCESS!©* *Series* titled *Assessing the Value of the Medical Practice.*

Basic to valuing a practice is to identify the intangible assets. Those assets include the following:

- Affiliation agreements

- Agreements (general)

- Book libraries

- Buy-sell agreement

- Certificates of need

- Computer software

- Computerized databases

- Contracts

- Cooperative agreements

- Employment contracts

- Expertise

- Favorable financing

- Favorable leases

- Goodwill

- HMO enrollment lists

- Laboratory notebooks

- Leasehold estates

- Location value

- Management contracts

- Manual databases

- Marketing and promotional materials

- Medical charts and records

- Noncompete covenants

- Procedural manuals

- Referral networks and relationships

- Regulatory approvals

- Reputation

- Technical and speciality libraries

- Technical documentation

- Trained and assembled workforce

- Trademarks and trade names

- Training manuals

A variety of conditions must be met regarding intangible assets, and all practices may not meet the criteria for all of the listed items.

The following generally do not qualify as identifiable intangible assets:

- High market share of the practice

- High profitability of the practice

- General positive reputation of the practice

- Monopoly position of the practice

- Market potential of the practice

- Other economic phenomena

Because of the multiple subjective and objective issues in determining the value of a practice to a seller and a buyer, first determine why you are doing the valuation and what use you plan to make of the outcomes. The value of the practice is often a difficult issue for attempting to satisfy both parties. Thus, the independent valuation by the physicians may prove to be a wise investment. Valuations are costly and require significant time from your current accounting firm and your practice administrator. Also understand the potential buyer, in all likelihood, will want to conduct his own valuation prior to purchase. He will want a full due diligence of the practice that includes the valuation of intangible assets and examination of a number of other issues such as the following:

- Compensation and benefits of physicians

- Compensation and benefits of staff

- Appraisals of real estate

- Physician and nonphysician production levels

- Physician recruitment expenses

- Accounts receivable analysis

- Third party agreements

- Current and future budgets

- Patient visits by provider

- Active charts by provider

- Numerous other documents and agreements

Key to a valid analysis will be strong communication between those conducting the valuation and those who actually operate and work in the practice. It is common for the records to only tell part of the story. Be sure you are kept up-to-date with any assumptions made and that you fully understand the process.

Strategically Selecting the Correct Partner for You and Your Practice

If you decide to partner—and the current thinking would suggest you should at some point— you should make your best judgement regarding choosing a partner. The following should help you with that determination:

- With your partners, create a vision statement for what role you want to play in the health care delivery system. Look at the options available to you and determine which one best matches your personal vision.

- Carefully explore your options including the following:
  - Access to patients
  - Physician compensation and benefit plans
  - Requirements to belong
  - Penalties for terminating
  - The organizational structure
  - The long term balance of your goals and those of your potential partners

- Reference all parties
  - Potential management
  - Physicians in leadership positions
  - Review others in the proposed partnership
  - Know the referral base
  - Review the financial strength of the organization(s).

- Understand your market
  - Gather and analyze data
  - Study local and national legislative issues
  - Contact colleagues in other markets and learn from them
  - Stay in close contact with MCOs and large employers in your region
  - Do not lose site of potential competitors to include nonphysician providers.

- Know your practice
  - Perform an independent analysis of your strengths, weaknesses, opportunities and threats
  - Understand the value of your practice in financial, geographic and service terms
  - Determine how your practice "fits" into the current market and how adaptable it is to future demands

- Know yourself
  - How do you want to practice?
  - How realistic are your choices?
  - Will your professional goals be met?
  - Is your style compatible with the organizational structure(s) you are considering?
  - Is your practice committed to being part of the solution?

Selection of a partner is a difficult decision. The odds are, however, the organization(s) you join or affiliate with today will look much differently two to five years from now. Be sure you have the level of involvement in these changes, in the transformation of your practice and the delivery system to create a solution that serves your interests and those of the patients you serve.

Addendum

Some Legal and Tax Considerations

Nothing can substitute in this environment for the services of an experienced health care attorney and an experienced health care accounting firm. The information below is not meant to provide advice, but rather to highlight some issues.

- Tax exempt status is afforded many health care organizations who are organized under not-for-profit state laws and have received a 501(c)(3) designation from the Internal Revenue Service. In exchange for that status, the benefits accorded to the community exceed the revenue the community could generate from taxes. In this type of organization, none of the net earnings may be distributed to any person or corporation except in exchange for bona fide services. To distribute these funds otherwise would be termed private inurement.

  Tax exempt status is not always the most attractive organizational structure. The pros and cons of each arrangement should be explored.

- Stark I law prohibits physicians from referring Medicaid or Medicare patients to clinical laboratories with which physicians have financial relationships subject to exemption.

- Stark II prohibits physicians from referring Medicare or Medicaid patients receiving "designated health services" to clinical laboratories, with which the physicians have financial relationships, again, subject to exemption.

- HMOs and insurers are subject to state insurance codes and statutes.

- Securities are subject to registration and disclosure requirements under federal and state law.

- Liability issues should be fully reviewed.

- Antitrust laws are stringent and applicable within local and regional markets.

Bibliography

Allevato, John. "Making sense of managed care models." *Unique Opportunities* (Jan./Feb. 1996): 9-13.

Aston, Geri. "Financial conflicts strain alliances." Vol. 31, *AHA News* (Apr. 24, 1995): 5.

Asplund, Jon. "Moody's urges caution." *AHA News* (May 20, 1996): 6.

Bledsoe, et al. "Practice acquisition: A due diligence checklist." Vol. 49, *Healthcare Financial Management* (Dec. 1, 1995): 36.

Braun, Joseph. "MSOs: Key to PHOs and community-based health care systems." Vol. 21, *Physician Executive* (Feb. 1, 1995): 28.

Cerne, Frank. "Money and management." Vol. 69, *Hospitals & Health Networks* (Jan. 5, 1995): 33.

David, R. "Caremark to acquire southland group; Mergers: Illinois-based firm will absorb Friendly Hills Healthcare Network in a deal worth more than $100 million." Home Edition, *Los Angeles Times* (Aug. 16, 1994): D-2.

Denscombe, Martyn. "The healthcare glossary." Vol. 88, *Southern Medical Journal* (May 1, 1995): 4.

Dube, Monte. "Restructuring public hospitals to meet marketplace demands." Vol. 50, *Healthcare Financial Management* (Feb. 1, 1996): 38.

Gawlick, Gerald. "Today's physician has choices, but needs help." Vol. 22, *Physician Executive* (Feb. 1, 1996): 24.

Green, J. "The Cost of Hospital Mergers." *Modern Healthcare* (Feb. 3, 1992): 36.

Hagland, Mark. "Anything but academic." Vol. 70, *Hospitals & Health Networks* (Jan. 1, 1996): 20.

Harris, Richard. "Models for medical practice integration." Vol. 20, *Physician Executive* (Aug. 1, 1994): 18.

Hickey, Martin. "From managing access to managing care: The impact of primary care on health care delivery." Vol. 21, *Physician Executive* (Oct. 1, 1995): 7.

Hill, John E., MBA, and Wild, Jennifer, MS. "Survey provides data on practice acquisiton activity." Vol. 49, *Healthcare Financial Management* (Sept. 1, 1995): 54.

Hodge, Robert. "The evolving role of the primary care physician." Vol. 20, *Physician Executive* (Oct. 1, 1994): 15.

Hudson, Terese. "Growing pains." Vol. 69, *Hospitals & Health Networks* (Jan. 5, 1995): 42.

Hurd, Douglas. "Benefits of group practice." Vol. 3, *Presidents & Prime Ministers* (May 1, 1994): 44.

Kerns, Eleanor H., CFA, Ockers, Nancy T. "Physician practice management industry: options facing physicians." Alex. Brown (Jan. 11, 1996).

King, Jeffrey. "Legal issues affecting IPA formation." Vol. 49, *Healthcare Financial Management* (Nov. 1, 1995): 24.

Kleiman, Mitchell. "Provider integration: PO versus PHO." Vol. 49, *Healthcare Financial Management* (June 1, 1995): 22.

Koeppen, Linda L., FACHE, RN, MHA, et al. "Effective planning for managed care." Vol. 49, *Healthcare Financial Management* (Nov. 1, 1995): 44.

Litle, Karen. "Essential ingredients for successful physician organizations (POs)." Vol. 89, *Southern Medical Journal* (Mar. 1, 1996): 3.

Louiselle, Paul. "Conducting financial due diligence of medical practices." Vol. 49, *Healthcare Financial Management* (Dec. 1, 1995): 28.

Lumsdon, Kevin. "How markets evolve." Vol. 69, *Hospitals & Health Networks* (Mar. 5, 1995): 48.

Mosvovice, Ira, Ph.D., et al. "Rural hospital networks: Implications for rural health reform." Vol. 17, *Health Care Financing Review* (Sept. 1, 1995): 53.

Peregrine, M. "Choosing medical practice acquisition models." Vol. 49, *Healthcare Financial Management* (Mar. 1, 1995): 58.

Pitta, Julie. "Doctor networks to merge in deal valued at $2.5 Billion; Health care: MedPartners/Mullikin's acquisition of Caremark would create the second-largest physicians group active in Southern California." *Los Angeles Times* (May 15, 1996): D-1.

Postman, Lore. "Physician-run network signs up payer groups." Vol. 16, *Indianapolis Business Journal* (Nov. 27, 1995): 4-A.

Rabe, James G., CFA, ASA, and Reilly, Robert F., ASA, CPA, CFA, CRA. "Looking beneath the surface valuing health care intangible assets." Vol. 41, *National Public Accountant* (Mar. 1, 1996): 14.

Robertson, Kathy. "It's becoming a doc-eat-doc world." Vol. 13, *Sacremento Business Journal* (June 17, 1996): 19.

Ross, Jon. "Houston." Vol. 69, *Hospitals & Health Networks* (May 5, 1995): 48.

Sachs, Laura. "The managed care answer book." Vol. 88, *Southern Medical Journal* (May 1, 1995): 3.

Sandrick, Karen. "How to succeed with doctors by really trying." Vol. 70, *Hospitals & Health Networks* (Jan. 1, 1996): 22.

Smith, Brian J., et al. "Financial options for integration." Vol. 48, *Trustee* (Jan. 1, 1995): 17.

Tucci, Linda. "AHA stats verify network expansion." Vol. 4, *Materials Management in Health Care* (Mar. 1, 1995): 80.

Wimp, Marilyn. "Bids accelerate for the region's physician practices." Vol. 15, *Philadelphia Business Journal* (June 14, 1996): 16-B.

Wolfson, Jay. "Overcoming challenges to tax-exempt status." Vol. 50, *Healthcare Financial Management* (Apr. 1, 1996): 58.

Zeff, Patricia. "Guide outlines physicians' new roles in future health systems." Vol. 31, *AHA News* (Oct. 30, 1995): 6.

Zismer, Daniel K., and Fansler, Davis D. "Valuing the primary care patient base." Vol. 25, *Minnesota Medicine* (Sept. 1993): 43-45.

Resources

Allina Health System: *1995 Environmental Assessment* (See p.4).

Health Gain, Improving the Health of Communities Through Integrated Health Care; an environmental assessment of the health care system in the United States, 1995–2000. Prepared for the U.S. Health Care Sector by: Allina Health System, Deloitte and Touche LLP, V.H.A.

Innovative Financing—Investor Owned Medical Groups—The Mysteries Unveiled; Dennis Calvert, Senior Vice President, Medical Asset Management, Inc., Mesa, AZ.